The Hairy Bikie and Other Metacognitive Strategies

Jeffrey Baron Levi

The Hairy Bikie and Other Metacognitive Strategies

Implementing a Frontal Lobe Prosthesis for Those Whose Learning Is Compromised

Springer

Jeffrey Baron Levi
Bogan Psychological Centre
Bondi Junction, Australia

ISBN 978-3-030-46620-6 ISBN 978-3-030-46618-3 (eBook)
https://doi.org/10.1007/978-3-030-46618-3

Cover illustration: Original illustrations by Marie Widolf marietwidolf_@hotmail.com

This Springer imprint is published by the registered company Springer Nature Switzerland AG
The registered company address is: Gewerbestrasse 11, 6330 Cham, Switzerland

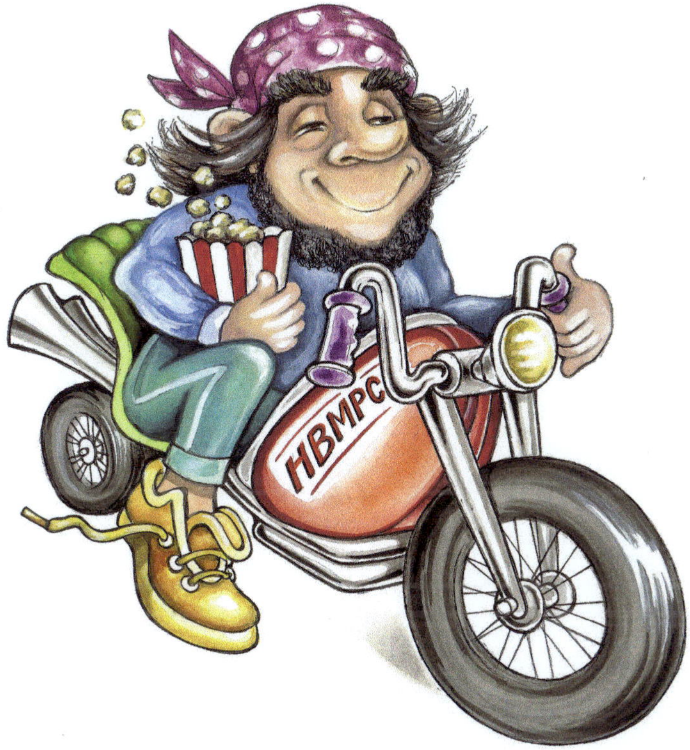
HBMPC

Foreword

To the uninitiated, making yourself familiar with the challenges specific to people living with brain injury may as well be like navigating Mars. For professionals seeking to build their capability in meeting those challenges, textbooks offering 'metacognitive strategies' might make their eyes glaze over or skip to the index. The unique difference in Jeffrey Baron Levi's approach is that it's rendered in plain English, with the kind of step-by-step guidance and adroit use of case studies that can only come from 30 years' worth of walking the talk everywhere from school classrooms to private practice.

Despite countless injury prevention campaigns, brain injury remains the leading cause of death in children and adolescents in high-income countries. While improvements in healthcare have meant that more survive initial injury, it is often at the cost of increased disability, with significant downstream impacts on education and family. The renewed focus on the potential protracted consequences of 'mild' brain injury has meant that only now are the true public health crisis and cost burden of the disability emerging.

Jeffrey's textbook is a 'one-stop-shop' as overdue as it is welcome: covering every aspect of the disability from general problem-solving, memory impairment, behaviour management to essay-writing and employment. I highly recommend it to any and all professionals and laypeople seeking to understand, and work with, people living with brain injury.

Executive Officer
Brain Injury Australia,
Marrickville, NSW, Australia

Nick Rushworth
nick.rushworth@braininjuryaustralia.org.au

Preface

For quite some years now, this book has been percolating through my cerebral system but a busy practice always seemed to impede its realisation. With 30 years of rehabilitation programs and strategies threatening to burst through my scalp, I decided it was finally time to put pen to paper or, at least, fingers to computer keys.

I would like to acknowledge the contribution and support of my beautiful wife Cheryl who worked with me over a number of years in providing rehabilitation to our clients. Cheryl's training and experience in special education, early intervention, administration and consultancy was invaluable in understanding the needs of our clients.

On a personal level, we could not have achieved what we did without her love and support and her belief in the work we were doing.

Sydney, Australia Jeffrey Baron Levi

Contents

About the Author

Jeffrey Baron Levi had a previous life as Jeffrey Bogan. He changed his name in November 2016. Dr Jeffrey Baron Levi holds the degrees of PhD from the University of New England and MA (Hons) and BA (Hons) both from the University of Sydney. He also has a Diploma of Teaching (NSW Department of Education) and the Certificate in Neuroanatomy for Neuropsychologists (University of NSW). Dr Baron Levi is a trained school counsellor having completed a full-time school counsellor training program. He taught in primary schools and worked as a school counsellor in schools in Australia and overseas providing assessment and counselling for children and adolescents with a range of issues including challenging behaviours and psychological issues. For several years, he coordinated special education services for the NSW Department of School Education in Western Sydney for students with a range of disabilities including Traumatic Brain Injury, Autism and ADHD and was the specialist counsellor for children with emotional and behavioural disorders.

He obtained his doctorate in neuropsychology on the assessment of executive function of young people with Traumatic Brain Injuries (TBI) as a consequence of a motor vehicle accident. Dr Baron Levi developed The Seals Test, a developmental measure of executive function and an adaptation of the Tower of Hanoi, and presented his findings at National and International Conferences of the International Neuropsychological Society, The Australasian Association of the Study of Brain Impairment and the College of Clinical Neuropsychologists.

Dr Baron Levi has had more than 35 years' experience in both assessment and rehabilitation of young people with psychological issues including anxiety, adjustment disorders and PTSD as well as TBI and Autism. Dr Baron Levi provided consultancy and individualised training to use compensatory strategies and support to young people and families who may have adjustment issues. Dr Baron Levi successfully conducted a 2-year research project funded by the NSW Motor Accidents Authority on training adolescents with TBI to improve their independence for learning in the classroom using metacognitive strategies. He has served on the National Steering Committee of the Head Injury Council of Australia examining services provided to students with TBI.

For 17 years, Dr Baron Levi was the director of a Disability Employment Service, which assisted jobseekers with a range of disability to find sustainable employment. He is currently the director of Toozly, a national recruitment website catering specifically for jobseekers with disability.

For the past 26 years, Dr Baron Levi has been conducting medico-legal assessments and cognitive rehabilitation for young people with trauma-related injuries including anxiety, adjustment issues, PTSD and TBI.

Dr Baron Levi has published several papers in the field of brain injury and self-esteem and has conducted workshops for teachers of students with TBI on behalf of the Queensland Brain Injury Association.

List of Figures

List of Tables

Chapter 1
Introduction

In 1989 I was coordinating special education services for the Metropolitan West Region of NSW Department of School Education in Australia and was aware that children who had sustained traumatic brain injuries from car accidents were being returned to schools after their physical recovery with little information to teachers on how to manage these students in the classroom. The first Paediatric Brain Injury Unit was established that year in Sydney at the Children's Hospital at Westmead. It was of concern that although these students appeared to look the same as before their accidents, they often presented with subtle learning and memory difficulties, disorganisation or behavioural problems. They were not the same students who were in the classroom before their accident. The majority of teachers did not know how to assist these students, many of whom may have spent weeks or months in hospital during their physical recovery.

When the brain injury unit was established around the middle of 1989, I immediately went about fostering a relationship with staff, and together we developed protocols for students involved in motor vehicle accidents to return to schools. It was important for teaching staff to have some knowledge of the impact of a brain injury on these vulnerable young students.

My task, as a special education coordinator for the region, was to take the clinical reports from hospital staff and translate these into instructionally designed programs to be used in the classroom to provide support to students and teachers during integration back into the school system. The issue was that although the clinical assessments by hospital neuropsychologists were useful in identifying areas of deficit, the clinical tests they used were never designed to yield usable information that was of assistance to school program designers or classroom teachers.

I began a journey of research and discovery that took me from developing specific strategies and protocols for students re-entering the school system following their recovery in hospital to developing specific strategies for teachers and students to compensate for student deficits. This culminated in 1994, in completing a PhD in the field of neuropsychology, focusing on executive functioning of children with

J. Baron Levi, *The Hairy Bikie and Other Metacognitive Strategies*,
https://doi.org/10.1007/978-3-030-46618-3_1

traumatic brain injury following an acceleration/deceleration injury such as a motor vehicle accident.

One Friday evening in 1993, my colleague and I were conducting a presentation for parents of students with traumatic brain injuries at the Children's Hospital at Westmead in Sydney. Mid-sentence she suddenly exclaimed that she did not feel well and collapsed on the stage. Doctors who were present quickly took her back to the emergency department, while I continued with the workshop.

At the conclusion of the presentation, I went back to see how she was doing, and she told me she had a bad headache. These were the last words she spoke. On Sunday her family reluctantly turned off the life support system. She was 42 years old, married with three young children and died of a cerebral aneurysm. The family asked me to give the eulogy at her funeral. It was a sobering and sad time for all of us who worked with her as she gave so much of herself to help children with traumatic brain injuries.

My colleague's death made me realise how short life can be and question what I really wanted to do with my working life. I believed that there was a lot more that could be done to assist young people with traumatic brain injuries. So I decided that what I really wanted to do was work exclusively with young people with traumatic brain injury without bureaucratic constraint. I resigned from the Department of Education at the end of that year and established a private practice providing cognitive rehabilitation on behalf of insurance companies for young people involved in motor vehicle accidents.

I first began experimenting with problem-solving strategies in 1991 and then refined them in 1994 while in private practice. I had an article published in an Australian magazine called THINK in December Baron Levi (1991), outlining the notion of a Problem Solving Plan to assist children with traumatic brain injuries to work independently in the classroom. A Problem Solving Plan was a kind of frontal lobe prosthesis. I had suggested in 1991 that "a plan can encompass the whole process of ensuring that the student knows what to do, what strategies to use in solving the problem, monitoring that the strategies are working, staying on task until the plan is completed and then verifying/rewarding yourself for successful completion".

The notion of a Problem Solving Plan was not only derived from a particular theoretical model of executive functioning and educational research but also represented an efficient teaching strategy.

My very first case in private practice was from an insurer who asked could I provide a program for a secondary student who was having anger issues in the classroom. He had suffered a traumatic brain injury as a result of a car accident and returned to his rural school some 600 km from Sydney. The problem was that as I was an untried entity; they asked if I could do the program remotely via telephone! It was not ideal to provide an intervention program in this manner, and I would not normally recommend it. However, I sent off my functional executive scale for teachers to complete, as well as a pro forma for observation of behaviours of concern, read all of the medical information and results of neuropsychological assessments and launched into developing a metacognitive strategy. I spoke to the boy's parents by phone as well as the school counsellor and obtained as much information as I could from them.

Once I had developed the plan, I spoke at length with the school counsellor who had previously agreed to coordinate the school program and carefully detailed how the strategies were to be implemented, the roles of the class teachers and how she was to present the program to the student. I coached the counsellor on ways she was to support the class teachers. I kept in regular contact with the counsellor over the following 2 weeks while the program was being implemented.

Miraculously, the program worked! This was my first case and it was a success. I continued to monitor the program over the following 2 months.

After that case the insurance companies had some confidence in me and prepared to send me off to work in situ with their clients. I was flown all around the state to see clients and even to places such as Germany and London to follow up on clients who had their accidents in Australia.

What I have learned over the past 25 years is that we are still only scratching the surface of discovering how to effectively teach those whose learning ability is compromised and how to compensate for their deficits so that they become efficient problem solvers. Ongoing research has provided support for the concept of neural plasticity and the notion that training individuals to use efficient metacognitive strategies Kolb et al (1998) also leads to positive changes in brain structure.

My motivation in writing this book was to impart some of the strategies that I have used successfully over the years in working with young people and adults with a wide range of disabilities including traumatic brain injury, ADHD and learning difficulties. Some of these strategies I had earlier presented at workshops and conferences, for example, the Hairy Bikie metacognitive strategy I presented at the International Neuropsychological Society Conference in Cairns, Australia, in July 1995.

I have used the problem-solving strategies with primary- or elementary-aged children, secondary and tertiary students and also adults in a range of settings. The youngest child I have worked with was 7 years of age. I have only a little experience working with preschool children. There are many special education and early intervention teachers who have been successfully using metacognitive-type strategies with preschool children.

This book is a product of the rehabilitation I have delivered between 1991 and 2018 to a range of clients with traumatic brain injuries, ADHD and learning disability in schools, universities and work settings. Through those years I developed numerous Problem Solving Plans, most of them for particular students or employees in particular situations. A Problem Solving Plans can be unique, or it can be generic, depending upon the circumstances. Every Problem Solving Plan was delivered in the student's or client's context or environment. In most cases I worked in the classroom, university, TAFE or workplace, teaching the individual to apply the processes to real problems. I also trained classroom teachers and employers to prompt their students or employees to use the strategies, and in many cases the plans were adapted to use with other students or employees. I ran workshops on behalf of the Queensland Brain Injury Association to a wide range of teachers and counsellors who were dealing with students with traumatic brain injuries. I also received regular referrals from Brain Injury Australia to provide consultancy to clients in a work setting.

I have explained some of the theory and research behind my approaches and given a brief summary of these at the end of each chapter. You will find the theoretical background to my strategies in Part I: Chapter 1 is the Introduction. Chapter 2 explains the concept of process-based learning which was the starting point for the development of my Problem Solving Plans. Chapter 3 examines the notion of executive function, while Chapter 4 explores the relationship between various disability groups and executive dysfunction. In Chap. 5, Part II, we finally arrive at the core of this book, which deals with the more practical aspects of metacognitive strategies. Chapter 6 addresses the notion of assessment where I include a Functional Executive Scale that I developed as a means of identifying various functional aspects of executive functioning. The remaining chapters deal with the very practical application of metacognitive strategies to a range of learning issues including problem solving, essay writing, memory, anger management and employment-related issues. I have included in Chap. 13 an abbreviated version of the research project I conducted to test the efficacy of the Hairy Bikie problem solving plan.

Feel free to skip Part I, the theoretical component, and dive straight into the practical strategies in Part II, although I always like to know how you arrive at particular rehabilitation approaches.

So, this book is an attempt to blend theory with practice in such a way that it will be readable to a wide group of professionals including teachers, rehabilitation consultants and psychologists as well as parents and those for whom this information will be new.

References

Baron Levi, J. (1991). Return to school: The integration of children with closed head injuries. *Think, The Australian magazine on acquired brain damage, 2*(1), 32–34.

Kolb, B., et al. (1998). Brain plasticity and behaviour. *Annual Review of Psychology, 49*, 43–64.

Part I
Introduction & Theoretical Background to Executive Function and Metacognition

Chapter 2
Process-Based Learning

The notion of applying metacognitive strategies to students came out of the work by two Australian researchers, Conway and Ashman (1989), who developed the concept of process-based instruction for students with intellectual disability. The students were taught to develop their own plans for specific curriculum content. The teacher would develop one plan for the class, and over time the students would develop their own plans using their own language. An example of a plan for writing was:

- Decide what the paragraph is about.
- Write sentences.
- Have you said what you want?
- Do your sentences relate to the idea?
- Are your sentences in the right order?

The researchers conducted a study involving students with mild intellectual disability and found significant increases in learning curriculum tasks using the structured curriculum plans compared to a matched control group.

According to Vermunt (1994), process-oriented instruction is defined as instruction aimed at teaching thinking strategies and domain-specific knowledge in coherence. The role of the teacher is to activate students' mental activities and their development of appropriate self-regulatory strategies for learning new content through modelling, cognitive coaching, guided learning and gradual transfer of control over learning processes to the student. Central to process-oriented instruction is the development of mental models and thinking strategies relevant to a particular field of study.

Dignath et al. (2008) defined self-regulated learning as process-based instruction and viewed self-regulated students as metacognitively, motivationally and behaviourally active participants in their own learning process. The authors cited three areas of psychological functioning in which self-regulated learning can appear: cognition, metacognition and motivation/affect.

J. Baron Levi, *The Hairy Bikie and Other Metacognitive Strategies*,
https://doi.org/10.1007/978-3-030-46618-3_2

Volet et al. (1995) concluded that instructional approaches involving structured forms of social interactions and guided learning were most effective for facilitating students' development of such strategies. The combination of metacognitive strategies enhancement and transfer of learning responsibility from an expert to a novice through modelling, coaching and reflective learning formed the essence of process-oriented instruction.

Naglieri and Johnson (2000) were of the view that some children performed poorly on mathematical problems because they did not apply appropriate methods when problem solving. They asserted that poor problem solving involved failure to organise the maths, inadequate reflection on the best procedures used, difficulty analysing the demands of the problem and failure to carefully monitor and check the work. Naglieri and Johnson proposed a new conceptualisation of cognitive processing based on the Planning, Attention, Simultaneous and Successive (PASS) theory. They claimed that all four of the PASS processes were statistically related to arithmetic computation.

The authors conducted a study using PASS with 19 students aged 12–14 who were placed in special educational settings for mathematics instruction. The results revealed that those students who had an identified weakness in Planning significantly improved following the intervention.

In a similar scenario, some university educators have moved away from a traditional lecture style to a problem-based learning approach with health science students Foord-May (2006). Problem-based learning used authentic clinical problems to address educational objectives. Workshops were offered by experts in problem-based instruction and included training in skills of questioning, active listening and guiding students' learning. The emphasis was on self-directed learning. Students worked in small groups working on authentic clinical cases. This approach taught students to structure their learning and organise information in ways that would be most useful to them in clinical practice.

The notion of process-based instruction in education involved both knowledge development and self-regulation of learning. It was the application of a metacognitive strategy to a particular content domain as in the case of the writing plan or in the teaching of complex mathematical concepts and involved modelling by an expert.

Meichenbaum and Biemiller (1998) used cognitive modelling and think-aloud strategies to teach skill acquisition to students. According to the authors, the actual demonstration component of an acquisition session usually involved both physically performing the skill or skills involved in the task and verbally guiding oneself (think out loud, demonstrate self-regulation overtly) while carrying out the task.

Think-alouds may be in the form of self-questioning (what information do I need? have I checked my work?) or self-instructional directive statements (My first step is.. This is not the answer I expected. I had better go back and re-check my steps). Think-alouds can describe the various steps of the problem-solving process and highlight the importance of each step.

Meichenbaum and Biemiller's concept of think-alouds were domain specific—they related to particular skill acquisition such as reading or writing. According to the authors, when writing a story, for example, the teacher would model the self-instructional technique. She may say: Let's look at an event—we'll say the school swimming carnival. Now, we'll say that David is the best swimmer in the school. The teacher writes the opening sentence. What do you think may happen to David when his turn to race in the carnival? The teacher encourages the class to brainstorm his ideas and together they choose one of the ideas.

In writing the story and modelling think-alouds, the following steps could be involved:

1. **Summarizing important information and planning**

   Let me see if I understand what I have to do?

2. **Accessing prior knowledge**

   What do I already know about this?
   How is this like what I have done before?

3. **Self-monitoring**

   How am I doing?
   Is this making sense?

4. **Accessing help**

   Who should I ask for help?

5. **Self-reinforcement**

   How did I do?
   I didn't get it all done, but I tried hard.

One of the major issues with process-based instruction or self-regulated learning was whether the skills taught in one situation would generalise or transfer to skills that were dissimilar. According to Meichenbaum and Biemiller, the absence of transfer by students of what they have learned is evident even on seemingly similar academic tasks. Unless students are prompted, they generally do not use what they have learned.

Through my reading and understanding of traumatic brain injury as well as my years of experience in special education with students with disabilities, I realised that the notion of process-based instruction or self-guided learning could be adapted to benefit students with traumatic brain injuries. Students with brain injuries, learning difficulty, autism spectrum disorder and attention deficit hyperactivity disorder (ADHD) essentially had difficulty with the processes of learning which were in fact executive in nature: they experienced difficulty with initiation of an activity, with sequencing, knowing and remembering what to do and then following through without being distracted.

My point of difference from the process-based instructional model or Meichenbaum's talk-aloud model was that I utilised a purely metacognitive strategy that could be applied across any particular content area. Unlike process-based instruction, a metacognitive strategy was content-free and simply involved a Problem Solving Plan that could be applied to any problem in any content domain.

The advantage of utilising a purely metacognitive strategy was that, as a generic problem solver, it could be applied to any content area and to any problem. The need to teach to generalisation or transfer of knowledge or skill becomes irrelevant.

I developed generic Problem Solving Plans, based on the processes of learning, which students could apply across all curriculum areas. Experimenting with different types of Problem Solving Plans over the years, I found that students were able to apply the strategies successfully and, after a period of reinforcement, internalise the steps. Teachers reported to me that they noticed improvements in the students' abilities to complete set work using the Problem Solving Plans. In effect, the Problem Solving Plans became a frontal lobe prosthesis.

At that time in 1990, the notion that you could teach strategies to students who had sustained a brain injury to overcome their deficits was completely foreign. The accepted wisdom from the brain injury community was that there was only a window of approximately 2 years of recovery following a brain injury and after that period of time there would be no further recovery of function.

In 1995 I was awarded a 2-year research grant funded by the then NSW Motor Accidents Authority to test the efficacy of the Hairy Bikie strategy that I had developed in 1993–1994. I had just completed my PhD in the field of neuropsychology on the developmental assessment of executive functions, and I was keen to conduct further research to test the veracity of the strategies that I had developed.

The project involved 42 adolescents with moderate traumatic brain injuries (TBI) as a result of motor vehicle accidents and who were studying in regular secondary schools in Sydney. There were three groups of students: a placebo group who received reading instruction, a second control group who received no instruction and the experimental group which received the direct instruction using the problem-solving plans applied to their school work. Students were randomly assigned to one of the groups, and each group was involved in the 20-week program.

The results revealed that the direct instruction group made significant improvements in their learning compared to the other groups, judging by teacher reporting on functional checklists of behaviour and also by direct observation. See Chap. 13 for a more detailed analysis of the research project.

I presented my Hairy Bikie metacognitive strategy at the International Neuropsychological Conference in Cairns, Australia, in July 1995 and continued to use that strategy and others which I had developed successfully over a period of 20 years with students in primary, secondary and tertiary institutions. I then applied the same processes to adults in work situations.

I consider that one of my greatest successes in using the Problem Solving Plan was with a university student who was run down by a car which mounted the footpath. He suffered a significant traumatic brain injury as a result. He was enrolled in Chemistry III Honours at the time. Following his recovery from the Brain Injury Unit, he returned to his studies which he failed. He failed a second year and was at the point of losing his place at the university. I became involved, successfully applied to the faculty dean for a continuance of his studies and worked one on one with him for a period of 12 months, initially in an intensive situation, and then gradually phased out my involvement. He failed to attend the first two sessions with me due to his general disorganisation, and my first task was to teach him diary skills to keep appointments.

I knew nothing about Chemistry Honours III, but I taught him metacognitive strategies to problem-solve his assignments and study routine. Fortunately, he was a very bright young man who was highly motivated to overcome his deficits. He successfully passed Chemistry III Honours that year using the problem-solving approach we developed together. By then he had internalised the strategies and successfully applied them to a range of problems. He went on to complete Chemistry IV Honours, successfully completed a PhD in Chemistry and was awarded a post-doctoral appointment overseas. I still have the letter of gratitude I received from his mother.

My interest in cognitive rehabilitation took a different turn when in 1996 I was invited to do some consultancy work to a disability employment service with their clients with traumatic brain injury. I began to experiment with my Problem Solving Plans with adults in a work setting. This was an entirely new field for me, and I began to investigate different models of supported employment. In 1998 I joined with this disability service in successfully securing a government contract to provide employment services for a range of clients with disability including those with TBI. We held the contract for 17 years and successfully placed hundreds of clients into new employment. As well I continued to provide individual consultancy to assist clients with TBI to secure new employment or return to work with the same employer.

Again, I would say a success story in this consultancy was to an employee who sustained a significant TBI in a motor vehicle accident while working overseas for the Australian government. He returned to his old job in Australia only to find that he struggled with anger management, disorganisation and distractibility. The organisation did not know what to do with him as he had difficulty coping with the demands of his old job. They provided him with work at a lower level, although he was not able to function on the job.

I became involved and spent time with him at home conducting various functional assessments and observing his behaviour in the home setting. It quickly became apparent that in the relaxed atmosphere at home, he had developed skills in gardening and had problem-solved some issues with birds that were attacking his fruit. I asked him how he came up with the ingenious idea, and he told me that he had done some reading on the internet and then adapted a particular method to his problem. Despite his poor results on neuropsychological testing of executive function, this man had demonstrated that in the real world, he had intact adaptive functioning! I could build on this skill.

I went back to his employer, and together with the client, we developed a program of guided return to work with support from mentors. The central part of the plan was using a Problem solving Plan which was developed in collaboration with the client and which would be reinforced by mentors in the workplace. He returned to work at a lower employment level to which he held prior to his accident with the view that if successful he could advance. I held regular meetings with his employer and mentors and helped them to problem-solve issues that arose. The client continued to successfully remain in employment.

References

Conway, R. N., & Ashman, A. F. (1989). Teaching planning skills in the classroom: The development of an integrated model. *International Journal of Disability, Development and Education, 36*(3), 225–240. University of Queensland Press.

Dignath, C., et al. (2008). Components of fostering self-regulated learning amongst students. A meta-analysis on intervention studies at primary and secondary school level. *Metacognitive Learning, 3*, 231–264.

Foord-May, L. (2006). A faculty's experience in changing instructional methods in a professional physical therapist education program. *Physical Therapy, Washington, 86*(2), 223–240.

Meichenbaum, M., & Biemiller. (1998). *Nurturing independent learners: Helping students take charge of their learning*. Cambridge, MA: Brookline Books.

Naglieri, J. A., & Johnson, D. (2000). Effectiveness of a cognitive strategy intervention in improving mathematical computation based on the PASS theory. *Journal of Learning Disabilities, 33*(6), 591–597.

Vermunt, J. D. H. M. (1994). Design principles of process-oriented instruction. In F. P. C. M. de Jong & B. H. A. M. van Hout-Wolters (Eds.), *Process-oriented instruction and learning from text* (pp. 15–26). Amsterdam: VU University Press.

Volet, S., et al. (1995). Implementing process-based instruction in regular university teaching: Conceptual, methodological and practical issues. *European Journal of Psychology of Education, 4*, 385–340.

Chapter 3
Compromised Learning Ability

Students, who suffer a traumatic brain injury (TBI); have attention deficit hyperactivity disorder (ADHD), conduct disorders (CD) or intellectual disability; have significant learning difficulties; or are diagnosed on the autism spectrum disorder (ASD), generally present with similar problems in learning. Their ability to carry out the following activities is often compromised:

- Follow a school timetable.
- Arrive at class with the correct materials.
- Know how to get started on set activities.
- Know and remember what they have to do.
- Stay on task without being distracted.
- Complete activities on time.
- Cope with changes in routine.

These behaviours are mediated by executive functions and pose serious constraints on the person's ability to function within a learning environment.

What Are Executive Functions and How Are They Developed?

For many years neuropsychologists have been debating the definition of executive functions Hass et al (2014). Even the basic question of whether executive function is a unitary process or a multifaceted construct is undecided. Some researchers believe that the term "executive function" is simply a heterogenous list of processes presumed to underlie performance.

Notwithstanding, the approach that I take is that executive functions are indeed a complex multifaceted concept that involves two related sets of abilities. According to Adilia (2008), one set of abilities relates to metacognitive functions which involve

J. Baron Levi, *The Hairy Bikie and Other Metacognitive Strategies*,
https://doi.org/10.1007/978-3-030-46618-3_3

planning, working memory and strategy development and implementation. The second set of abilities coordinates cognition and emotion to follow socially acceptable strategies. This second set of abilities is about emotional regulation of behaviour and is particularly compromised in young people on the autism spectrum disorder.

The term "executive function" is often used interchangeably with frontal lobe functions and, in particular, the prefrontal cortex. The prefrontal cortex is the association cortex of the frontal lobe and is located at the front of the frontal lobe. It is one of the last brain structures to develop in the course of evolution. In humans, it constitutes more than one-quarter of the entire cerebral cortex. Research on patients with frontal lobe damage has shown that they often have difficulty with tasks defined as "executive" in nature, including maintaining self-control, shifting attention, planning, organising, solving problems and making decisions.

The prefrontal cortex is indeed the executive of the brain and has connections to all brain functions except the sense of smell. In a sense you can visualise the executive functions as the conductor of an orchestra—it orchestrates and controls most of our brain functioning toward goal-directed behaviour. So, it is critical to everyday adaptive behaviour.

In an acceleration/deceleration injury in a motor vehicle accident or a fall, the brain is rotated inside the skull causing brain matter to shear. This is most evident in the frontal and occipital lobes as the brain moves back and forward inside the bony sections of the skull. The result is diffuse axonal damage (white matter connections), with a slowing of brain function and subtle frontal lobe or executive function impairment.

Figure 3.1 is a diagram showing the various lobes of the brain and their reported functions. You can see that the functions of the prefrontal cortex are critical to learning. All of the prefrontal cortex functions that we are currently aware of are essential to development, to learning and to adaptive functioning. Other functions from different lobes also come into play and are integrated into performance of a particular task which may be essentially executive in nature. For example, the functions of the temporal lobe in terms of language and memory are critical to the performance of executive functioning. As in the conductor of an orchestra, the prefrontal cortex can call into play all relevant sections of the brain to produce a desired and harmonious outcome.

So, we know that according to Finnager et al. (2015), executive function is a complex, overarching concept that refers to all functions related to goal-directed regulation of thoughts, actions and emotions, including problem-solving, monitoring ongoing operations, switching between operations, emotion regulation, initiation of behaviour, working memory, mental flexibility and inhibition of non-adaptive behaviour. It is independent of general intelligence. There are examples in the literature of very bright academics who suffered a TBI and, despite maintaining their high intellectual status, had difficulty carrying out simple everyday tasks such as making a cup of tea because of lack of problem solving and sequencing abilities as a result of frontal lobe damage.

According to Garcia et al. (2014), executive functions involve a series of cognitive, behavioural and affective-emotional components, which play an important role in regulating and organising one's behaviour in a wide range of situations, especially in those that require a creative and novel approach.

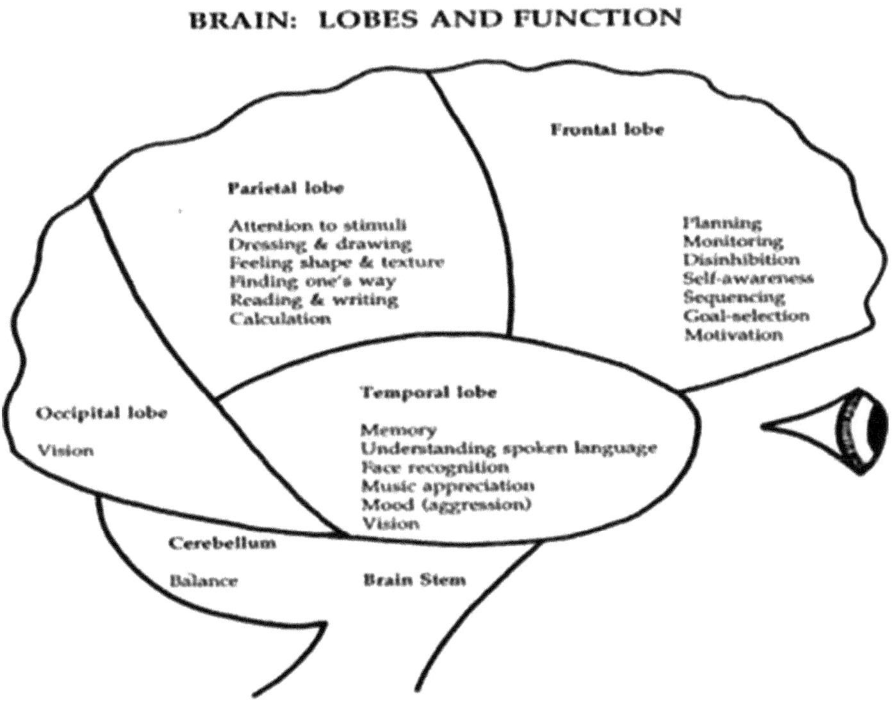

Fig. 3.1 Map of the brain and its functions with particular reference to prefrontal cortex

Executive functions come into play when a novel or complex problem presents itself or when a routine is disrupted. Think of driving to work every day. In the beginning you had to work out the most efficient way to get to work. You planned and problem-solved and tried different routes and different times of the day until you arrived at the quickest route. You eventually decided that leaving at a particular time in the morning and using the back roads, you avoided the traffic and the traffic lights and you arrived in the shortest time. Your executive functions mediated this type of problem-solving behaviour.

Then you travelled the same route every morning, and it became so routinised that you didn't even have to think about it. You were on auto-drive as it were. Some days you were puzzling over a problem or thinking about shopping after work or you were deep in thought, and suddenly you found that you had arrived at your destination! You didn't have to think about the way you went because it had become a routinised behaviour.

Now, what happened if during the same trip a car suddenly jumped out at you and was going to collide with you if you didn't take evasive action or there was roadwork and you had to take a detour? That was when your executive functioning stepped in again, quickly appraised the situation, weighed up the options and took appropriate action to either avoid a collision or find an alternate route.

Or, what happened if you learnt to drive on the left-hand side of the road as we did in Australia and you moved to Europe or the USA where you drove on the right-hand side? This was a whole new set of driving principles that you had to suddenly learn. For example, if you made a left-hand turn, your natural inclination would be to move to the left-hand side of the road! Enter your executive function processes to problem-solve.

I have always maintained that certain fast food chains or restaurants don't use their frontal lobes. You go into a restaurant and you ask for apricot nectar with a scoop of ice cream. The waitress informs you that they cannot do that as that item is not on the menu. You check the menu, and it clearly states that they serve apricot nectar, and over the page it states that they also have ice cream. You simply want the two together in one glass. "Sorry, we cannot provide that as that particular dish is not on the menu". So, you tell the waitress that you want the nectar in a glass, and she can serve the ice cream in a separate dish, and you will put the two together! Problem solved.

The waitress or the restaurant is inflexible in its approach to customers and not able to solve a simple problem that could be remedied easily. I am sure everybody at some time has encountered examples of inflexible approaches where a simple solution could have been found if only they had used their frontal lobes!

References

Adilia, A. (2008). On the evolutionary origins of executive functions. *Brain and Cognition, 68*, 92–99.

Finnager, T. G., et al. (2015). Life after adolescent and adult moderate and severe traumatic brain injury: Self-reported executive, emotional and behavioural function 2-5 years after injury. *Behavioural Neurology, 2015*, 329241. 1–19.

Garcia, T., et al. (2014). Executive functions and their assessment in children and adolescents. *Cognitive Sciences; Hauppauge, 9*(2), 101–116.

Hass, M., et al. (2014). Assessing executive functioning: A pragmatic review. *Contemporary School Psychology; Heidelberg, 18*(2), 91–102.

Chapter 4
Executive Functions (EF), Traumatic Brain Injury (TBI), Attention Deficit Hyperactivity Disorder (ADHD), Autism Spectrum Disorder (ASD), Conduct Disorder (CD) and Learning Difficulty (LD)

Prefrontal cortex impairment or executive function impairment can be the result of damage to the brain as in a traumatic brain injury or insult or immature development of the brain as in a developmental disorder. Although there are rough guidelines for typical development, it is important to keep in mind that brains mature at different rates and that individual differences result in considerable variability in functioning among children at any given age. In keeping with this, many of the specific abilities associated with executive functioning also appear to have different developmental trajectories.

There is evidence that the development of prefrontal cortex functioning mirrors cognitive development and those with learning difficulties, ADHD, conduct disorder (CD), ASD or intellectual impairment often have executive function deficits, not as the result of an injury but from immature development of the frontal lobes as in a developmental disorder.

According to Fuster (2002), the cognitive development of the child and adolescent appears to correlate with the development of the prefrontal cortex. This correlation is most obvious as we consider the evolution with chronological age of these cognitive functions of the prefrontal cortex that most contribute to intellectual maturation: attention, language and creativity. All depend on the ability to organise behaviour and cognition into goal-directed structures of action. According to Piaget (1971), the development of this ability follows certain trends through a series of well-defined stages and milestones.

After a first stage of simple sensory motor integration and primitive symbolisation, the child from 2 to 7 enters a representational stage of extended verbal symbolism. Language becomes progressively more elaborate and governed by external feedback, including language from other persons. The child learns to delay gratification in the next period from 7 to 11; language and behaviour become more structured, more independent of external stimuli and more creative. Problem solving becomes important. From 11 to 15 and beyond, the child begins to utilise logical reasoning for the construction of hypotheses and the testing of alternative solutions. Both induction and deduction become the means to do it. The adolescent becomes

J. Baron Levi, *The Hairy Bikie and Other Metacognitive Strategies*,
https://doi.org/10.1007/978-3-030-46618-3_4

progressively better capable of integrating information in the time domain and therefore more goal-directed. These developments continue into late adolescence and correspondence to full maturation of the prefrontal cortex.

There is comprehensive evidence from EEG studies from Thatcher (1992), which confirm these prefrontal cortex growth spurts at ages up to 5 years, 7–9 years, 11–13 years and 14–16 years. As Fuster opines, these same age spans correspond to Piagetian stages of cognitive development culminating in the period of formal operational reasoning involving hypothetico-deductive reasoning ability. The stage of formal operational reasoning marks the period of the ability to solve complex problems and generalise the results across different situations. The period between late concrete operational and early formal operational reasoning, where thinking and problem-solving processes move from one based on empirico-inductive to one based on more sophisticated hypothetico-deductive reasoning, represents one of those rapid periods in development.

However, not all adolescents and adults achieve the level of Piagetian formal operational reasoning.

In particular, children and adolescents with ADHD, conduct disorder, learning difficulty, autism spectrum disorder and intellectual disability often do not reach this level of cognitive development. Their deficits in executive functions are often the product of a neurodevelopmental disorder.

One interesting theory on the relationship between executive function and developmental disorders such as autism and attention deficit hyperactivity disorder was proposed by Johnson (2012). He acknowledged the evidence that the developmental disorders which emerge during early to middle childhood were associated with impairments in executive function. However, Johnson was of the opinion, contrary to the prevailing view, that, within populations at risk, the association with executive function was found because individuals with strong executive function skills were better able to compensate for atypicalities in other brain systems early in life and were therefore less likely to receive a diagnosis later in life. Johnson discussed evidence consistent with this view from considerations of individual variability, neuroimaging and genetics. To the extent that this view was correct, it offered hope for remediation of some later emerging symptoms, as evidenced from typical groups indicated that training programs for executive function in preschoolers may be effective in improving skills.

What evidence is there that children and adolescents with ADHD, learning difficulty, autism spectrum disorder, conduct disorder and Tourette syndrome have executive function deficits?

ADHD and Executive Function Deficits

Mahone et al. (2001) indicate that children with ADHD and Tourette syndrome have significant deficits with inhibition and fluency, two of the hallmarks of executive function. In one study, Cortese et al. (2013) opine that besides the behavioural core symptoms of inattention, hyperactivity and impulsivity, deficits in executive functions are commonly, although not universally, associated with ADHD. Weyandt (2009) concludes that ADHD is not a behavioural disorder but rather a cognitive disorder due to developmental impairment of executive functions.

Wilcutt et al. (2005) reported in a meta-analysis that children with ADHD tended to perform worse than children without the disorder on planning and organisational tasks, working memory and response inhibition but that their performance was not consistently impaired on executive function measures involving set-shifting or interference. There was also evidence from Weyandt and Colleagues (2009) that children with ADHD and either a reading disability or learning difficulty performed worse on measures of executive function than those with just a pure form of ADHD.

Autism Spectrum Disorder and Executive Function Deficits

According to Verte et al. (2005), autism is a lifelong developmental disorder with a triad of characteristic symptoms: (a) qualitative impairment in social interactions; (b) qualitative impairment in communication; and (c) stereotypic restricted, repetitive pattern of behaviour, interests and activities.

Winsler et al. (2007) observe that a large number of studies has identified that children with autism spectrum disorder (ASD) have particular difficulties with executive functioning, leading executive functioning to be one of the major theories of the core deficit present in autism. In particular, planning and cognitive flexibility are the two components of executive functioning most consistently reported to be impaired among autistic individuals.

Robinson and colleagues (2009) administered various tests of executive functioning to 54 children with ASD with a matched control group in a study. A multidimensional notion of executive functions was proposed, with difficulties in planning, the inhibition of prepotent responses and self-monitoring reflecting characteristic features of ASD that are independent of IQ and verbal ability and relatively stable across the childhood years.

Biro and Russell (2001) have shown that children with ASD have trouble specifically with executive tasks that require following arbitrary, novel rules (i.e. "if it is red, put it here") and those with nonverbal response modes. When executive tasks do not involve following arbitrary rules and/or when tasks require children to respond verbally, high-functioning autistic children do not appear to be impaired. The authors stated that tests on which executive functioning are assessed typically involve two components: (1) holding in mind task-relevant information while (2) inhibiting prepotent responses. They found that children with autism performed poorly on tasks that involved arbitrariness without prepotency as well as those with arbitrariness and prepotency. These demands were certainly present in tests such as the Wisconsin Card Sorting Test and the Tower of Hanoi.

Learning Difficulties and Executive Function Deficit

Researchers examining the relationship between learning difficulties and executive function conducted a study involving 23 students with learning difficulties and dyslexia. The results indicated that children with dyslexia had the worst performance on different measures of attention and executive functions, indicating that such changes may be characteristic of the disorder and keep the deficit in the phonological component of language.

Intact executive functions are critical to learning. There is evidence from Bull and Scerif (2001) that executive functions predict mathematical ability in children. In their research study, the authors concluded that children of lower mathematical ability displayed difficulties on tasks that measured the ability to inhibit both prepotent information and learned strategies; these children also had difficulty maintaining information in working memory.

In another study, Bental et al. (2007) involved 93 children with ADHD plus reading disorder and a group with just pure reading disorder and concluded that reading disorder was associated with deficits in working memory and rapid naming.

Conduct Disorders and Executive Function Deficit

DSM5 defines oppositional defiant disorder (ODD) as a recurrent pattern of negativistic, defiant, disobedient, and hostile behaviour toward authority figures. Conduct disorder is characterized by a repetitive and persistent pattern of behaviour in which the basic rights of others or major age-appropriate societal norms or rules are violated. Prateeksha et al. (2014) maintain that children with conduct disorders are known to be vindictive, frequently blame others for their mistakes and can be intentionally cruel to people and animals, indicating a lack of empathy. The authors conducted a study involving 13 children diagnosed with conduct disorder and a matched group of neurotypicals and found that the conduct disordered children performed significantly poorly on measures of response inhibition, a major component of executive functioning.

According to a study from Finland, Anon (2010) in group-level studies of adolescents with conduct disorder (CD) found deficiencies in verbal and executive functions. They were of the view that neuropsychological deficits should be taken into account in assessing and planning interventions for adolescents with conduct disorder.

Regarding the type of executive function impairment, Schoori (2018) reported various deficits such as working memory, cognitive flexibility and planning impairments or sustained attention and inhibition.

According to Matthys (2012), problem solving is impaired in children and adolescents with conduct disorders due to deficiencies in inhibition, attention, cognitive flexibility and decision-making. Consequently, children and adolescents with ODD and CD may have difficulty learning to optimize their behaviour in changeable environments.

Schoori et al. (2016) studied emotion regulation in boys with oppositional defiant disorder and conduct disorder as previous research had pointed toward a link between emotion dysregulation and aggressive behaviour in children. They argue that children with aggression problems have been found to be less likely to inhibit emotional reactivity and use less effective or more inappropriate regulatory strategies. In their study Schoori reported that boys with ODD/CD showed impaired emotional decision-making and emotion regulation in daily life but had reduced self-awareness. Their main point is that problems with emotion regulation in boys with ODD/CD lead to losing temper, irritability and being easily annoyed as a result of misinterpreted internal and external emotional cues. It is the inability to inhibit inappropriate strategies or responses in the face of this misinterpretation of emotional cues that leads to aggressive acts.

What Does This Mean?

The evidence from research studies confirms the consistent relationship between ADHD, learning difficulties, ASD, conduct disorders, obsessive-compulsive disorder, traumatic brain injury and executive function deficit. This deficit is the result either of impairment of the prefrontal cortex or of a development disorder of the prefrontal cortex. The majority of studies identified planning, working memory and organisational deficits as the executive dysfunction. These are the very skills that are required for effective learning and problem solving and clearly tie the various disability groups into possessing a similar profile in terms of a rehabilitation plan. There is evidence that emotional dysregulation of behaviour, lack of awareness of the emotion and the inability to inhibit inappropriate responses to the emotion are also driving forces behind ODD and CD.

I have worked with a range of young people with executive function impairment including problems with planning, working memory and organisational deficits. My experience is that teaching them to use metacognitive strategies is an effective method to overcome or compensate for difficulties in problem solving.

I am also of the view that like autism, there is a spectrum along which we all fit in terms of our capacity for executive functioning. This notion fits with the concept that executive function is a developmental process and that there are individual differences in the rate of development. It is because of this that many of the teachers whose students have a disability and with whom I have provided an intervention program often say to me that they have several students in their class who would also benefit from using metacognitive strategies. These students may be of average ability, do not present with a disability, although would benefit from the structure that metacognitive strategies offer. Often I am told that there are other students who are more needy than the targeted student.

Consequently, I tend to encourage the teachers that I have worked with to use the same metacognitive strategies with their class. I am always delighted when I return to the classroom to follow up on a particular student to find that the teacher has printed out a particular strategy in large print and placed it at the front of the classroom for all of her students to follow. This approach is also beneficial for the targeted student who doesn't feel singled out and "special".

References

Anon. (2010). Conduct disorder; Data on conduct disorder published by researchers at University of Jyvaskyla. *Psychology & Psychiatry Journal*; Atlanta: 80.

Bental, B., et al. (2007). The relationship between attention, executive function and reading domain abilities in attention deficit hyperactivity disorder and reading disorder: A comparative study. *The Journal of Child Psychology and Psychiatry, 48*(5), 455–463.

Biro, S., & Russell, J. (2001). The execution of arbitrary procedures by children with autism. *Development and Psychopathology, 13*, 97–110.

Bull, R., & Scerif, G. (2001). Executive functioning as a predictor of children's mathematics ability: Inhibition, switching, and working memory. *Developmental Neuropsychology, 19*(3), 273–293.

Cortese, S., et al. (2013). Attention deficit hyperactivity disorder. Impairment in executive functions: A barrier to weight loss in individuals with obesity. *BMC Psychiatry, 13*, 286–293.

Fuster, J. (2002). Frontal lobe and cognitive development. *Journal of Neurocytology, 31*(3), 373–385.

Johnson, M. H. (2012). Executive function and developmental disorders: The Flip side of the coin. *Trends in Cognitive Sciences, 16*(9), 454–457.

Mahone, E. H., et al. (2001). Executive function in fluency and recall measures among children with ADHD or Tourette. *Journal of the International Neuropsychological Society, 7*, 102–111.

Matthys, W., et al. (2012). Impaired neurocognitive functions affect social learning processes in oppositional defiant disorder and conduct disorder: Implications for interventions. *Clinical Child and Family Psychology Review, 15*, 234–246.

Piaget, J. (1971). The theory of stages in cognitive development. In D. R. Green, M. P. Ford, & G. B. Flamer (Eds.), *Measurement and Piaget*. New York: McGraw Hill.

Prateeksha, S., et al. (2014). Response inhibition in children with conduct disorder: A preliminary report. *Indian Journal of Health & Wellbeing, 5*(11), 1325–1330.

Robinson, S., et al. (2009). Executive functions in children with autism spectrum disorders. *Brain and Cognition, 71*(3), 362–368.

Schoori, J., et al. (2016). Emotion regulation difficulties in boys with oppositional defiant disorder/conduct disorder and relation to comorbid autism traits and attention deficit traits. *PLoS One*. https://doi.org/10.1371/journal.pone.0159323.

Schoori, J., et al. (2018). Boys with oppositional defiant disorder/conduct disorder show impaired adaptation during stress: An executive functioning study. *Child Psychiatry and Human Development, 49*, 298–307.

Thatcher, R. W. (1992). Cyclic cortical reorganisation during early childhood. *Brain and Cognition, 20*, 24–50.

Verte, S., et al. (2005). Executive functioning in children with autism and Tourette syndrome. *Development and Psychopathology, 17*(2), 415–445.

Weyandt, L. L. (2009). Executive functions and attention deficit hyperactivity disorder. *The ADHD Report New York, 17*(6), 1–7.

Wilcutt, E. G., et al. (2005). Neuropsychological analyses of comorbidity between reading disability and attention deficit hyperactivity disorder. In search of the common deficit. *Developmental Neuropsychology, 21*, 35–78.

Winsler, A., et al. (2007). Private speech and executive functioning among high-functioning children with autistic spectrum disorders. *Journal of Autism and Developmental Disorders, 37*, 1617–1635.

Part II
From Theory to Practice: The Metacognitive Strategies

Chapter 5
Metacognitive Strategies

Promoting metacognitive and executive skills has increasingly become a focus in head injury rehabilitation for both children and adults. My view is that rehabilitation should focus on the processes of learning by providing structured metacognitive activities designed to teach compensatory strategies (Baron Levi 1995). In this way the strategies can be applied across any content area as the processes of learning remain the same whether you are studying chemistry or history or planning a holiday.

What Are Metacognitive Strategies?

Metacognitive activities include planning how to approach a learning task, using appropriate skills and strategies to solve a problem, monitoring one's own comprehension of text, self-assessing and self-correcting in response to the self-assessment and evaluating progress toward the completion of a task. It is about *learning how to learn* and in particular the most effective way for an individual to learn. There is a close relationship between metacognitive functioning and executive functioning. Both involve planning, memory, organisation and cognitive flexibility to control the processes of learning.

There are generally two components to metacognition: metacognitive knowledge and metacognitive skills. Metacognitive knowledge refers to knowledge about oneself as a learner or problem solver. For example, are you more a visual or a verbal learner? Maybe you use both processes. When I am learning a new mobile phone number, for example, I visualise the first component and then verbalise the second until I can write it down or plug it into my phone. If you are mainly a verbal learner, then perhaps you self-rehearse the information you are learning until it is captured into your memory system.

J. Baron Levi, *The Hairy Bikie and Other Metacognitive Strategies*,
https://doi.org/10.1007/978-3-030-46618-3_5

Metacognitive skill, on the other hand, according to Garcia (2016), refers to higher-order skills and involves a component of regulation of one's own cognition and behaviour.

When I was studying and needed to learn a complex set of principles, I would write down the main components of each principle that I needed to learn and identify a keyword within each component that would jog my memory, maybe even the first letter of that component. I would then arrange each letter or word into a meaningful anagram or sentence and remember that mnemonic. Then when I needed to apply the set of principles, I would recall the mnemonic and unpack it.

For example, to recall the frontal subcortical circuitry, I would write out the important information. The circuitry involved three cortical regions: dorsolateral, ventromedial and orbitofrontal. I needed to remember the functions of each of these regions for a Psychology II assessment, so I wrote them out, used the first letter of each function and arranged the letters into a word or a nonword that I could remember. For example, with the dorsolateral region, I came up with the mnemonic "paws" which stood for planning, abstract thinking, working memory and shift set.

We can all recall the sentence we learned to identify the planets in our solar system. Perhaps you used the following: "My very enthusiastic mother just served us noodles". Or when remembering the treble clef lines for the piano (EGBDF) "Every good boy deserves fruit".

In fact, the problem solving plan that I will discuss later in Chap. 7 is predicated on learning a mnemonic: Hairy Bikie Munches Pop Corn (HBMPC).

As learners we often experiment to determine the most effective method to learn—it may not come naturally to us at first. How do you work out the best way to learn? Do you just stumble on it or trial and error or do you have an epiphany? When I was in Psychology 1 at the university, I read that the brain is most receptive to learning just before REM sleep. So, in preparation for an examination, I recorded on my tape recorder all of the basic information I needed to remember and then spliced the tape into a loop. This was in the 1960s when my parents bought me a reel-to-reel tape recorder, and then I played that loop all night until I fell asleep. Of course, when I woke up, I was tired and could recall nothing of the information I needed to learn! This was not the method for me.

Metacognitive and executive function learning processes include attending, concentrating, planning and problem solving. According to Ylvisaker (1994), this approach involves an instructional focus of self-awareness of needs, realistic goal-setting, planning, self-initiating and self-monitoring. The notion of rehabilitation is to provide structured metacognitive strategies designed to teach compensatory strategies. These structured activities are viewed as executive in nature and provide a type of frontal lobe prosthesis.

There is a rich developmental literature on treatment programs for children and adolescents with a wide range of disabilities and learning difficulties using a metacognitive approach. Meichenbaum (1977) trained hyperactive children to improve their level of attention by employing a verbal self-instructional program. The trainer first talked through the task with the child using a sequence of metacognitive instructions and gradually taught the child to use the same instructions to modulate their own attention and behaviour.

I recall attending an international conference where Dr Mark Yvilsaker talked about training adolescents with behaviour problems to teach themselves strategies to control their behaviour by videotaping themselves being the trainer. Dr Yvilsaker talked through the approach the adolescents would take in being their own trainers—the language of encouragement they should use. He then videotaped the adolescents talking to themselves and encouraging themselves to apply the strategies they had been taught. The adolescents then played the tapes to themselves every night: they became their own coaches reminding themselves of the strategies they should use, how to avoid anger inducing situations and how to deal with them. The program was successful in mitigating anger.

After experimenting with the use of video recording of clients, I began using photographs of clients engaged in a sequence of activities as a form of Problem Solving Plan. These clients typically would confuse a particular sequence of activities. One client who had a significant traumatic brain injury would confuse the sequence of clothing she needed to put on in order to dress herself. My wife worked with her and took a photo of each garment that the client wore and then arranged the photos in the correct sequence and placed these on a chart which was kept in the client's bedroom. After a short period of prompting, the client managed to successfully dress herself referring to the sequence of photos on the chart.

I then used the same method with a client who had started a work trial at a veterinary clinic. His part-time job was to clean out the enclosures for the animals each morning and then to feed the animals, ensuring that they had fresh water each morning. The activities involved the same routine each morning. I took a photo of my client engaged in each activity and placed the photos on a chart which hung on the wall adjacent to the animal enclosures.

I then worked each morning with my client, prompting him to check the sequence of activities after he had successfully completed each activity. He eventually internalised the routine and was able to complete his work trial (Fig. 5.1).

Marulis et al. (2016) assert that metacognitive strategies can be taught to children as young as 3 years of age. They were able to detect evidence of contextualised metacognition in 3–5-year-old preschool children through the use of observational assessment tools. Lyons and Ghetti (2010) concluded that young children may be much more adept at monitoring their mental activity than is often assumed. Marulis opined that the origins of metacognition may be present in infants as young as 2–4 months of age at which time they begin to be able to participate in joint monitoring and control interactions with adults.

Interestingly, Whitebread et al. (2009) developed a checklist of metacognitive behaviours for 3–5-year-olds, in the form of an observational instrument, the Children's Independent Learning Development (CHILD 3–5). I believe the CHILD has much in common with the functional executive scale (FES) which I developed for older children in that it is contextualised within the child's environment. See Chap. 6 on assessment for details on the FES.

For many years early childhood teachers have been successfully using metacognitive strategies with preschoolers. Children on the autism spectrum disorder, for example, are being identified at earlier ages, in some cases around 2 years of age.

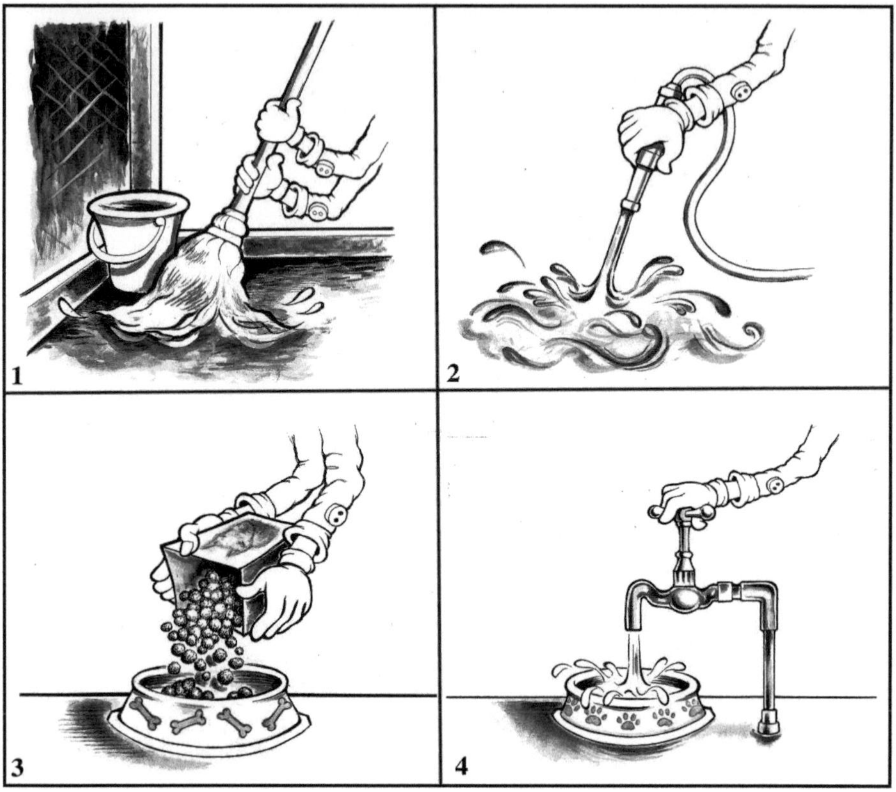

Fig. 5.1 The sequence of photos shows the various tasks that my client was required to perform each day. I placed them in the sequence in which he was required to carry out each task and placed them on a chart which we kept in his allotted area

Often these children initially present as having behavioural issues and are misdiagnosed as having ADHD.

The plan would be to keep the steps in any problem solving plan as simple as possible and to use pictures or icons rather than words.

With young children on the autism spectrum or with behavioural problems, it is often the case that they place themselves in dangerous situations as they are not aware of the consequences of their behaviour or the imminent danger of a particular action.

Cheryl and I worked with a 4-year-old who was diagnosed with autism. He had a habit of running off and not waiting for his caregivers to take him out. He would hurriedly put on his shoes and without waiting for an adult would be out the door. If the caregiver happened to be getting herself ready and not watching the child, she could easily have lost him on a number of occasions.

We encouraged the caregiver to use very simple language as an instruction and then the full sentence. In this way the child was given just the main words/concepts so that he was not immediately overwhelmed with a lot of superfluous language. Then he was given the full sentence because that was eventually going to be the instruction we wanted him to understand. The caregiver said to him "First shoes, then park", and then she would say "Put your shoes on and then we go to the park". Of course, what we wanted our 4-year-old to do was to put on his shoes and wait at the door for the caregiver to be ready to take him to the park. We printed a large red stop sign and placed it on the front door and showed the child, saying: "STOP!", holding out our hand in a stop position and saying "No go!". The caregiver did this over a period of several days. Then we combined the steps by putting together the sequence of "first shoes then stop at door". We noted that after a short period of time, our 4-year-old quickly learned the sequence. We did observe that after he had put on his shoes and went to the front door, he looked at the STOP sign and then turned around to his caregiver, presumably to gain acknowledgement that he was complying. Then the caregiver took him out to the park.

Our 4-year-old quickly learned to stop at the door, although after 2 weeks of successfully following the sequence, he regressed and actually ran out the door without waiting. The caregiver understood that she would need to keep reinforcing the sequence and eventually he would internalise the sequence.

As an early intervention support teacher, Cheryl introduced various sequence charts to guide the children in learning routines or understanding what would be happening. The arrival routine photo chart was displayed in the locker area, where each child had an open locker cupboard. This would be a set routine each day. Initially, verbal instructions would be given as appropriate while pointing to the appropriate picture. The instructions would be faded out, initially prompting the child to look at the chart, as necessary for the next instruction. Very quickly the children were able to follow the sequence without guidance (Fig. 5.2).

Through the application of a metacognitive strategy, are we compensating for a deficit, or are we restoring a function? This question raises the issue of whether the notion of neural plasticity is a reality. Is the brain malleable so that it can regenerate structure?

Do Metacognitive Strategies Have the Capacity to Change the Structure of the Brain?

The simple answer is yes! There have been a large number of studies now which demonstrate that strategic training can increase grey matter volume and cortical thickening and that these changes significantly and positively alter the functioning of the individual in the long term. There are basically two types of cognitive and behavioural rehabilitation: restorative training focuses on improving a specific cognitive function, whereas compensatory training focuses on adapting to the presence of a cognitive deficit. Some programs rely on a single strategy such as computer-assisted cognitive training; others use an integrated strategy which can be both restorative and compensatory.

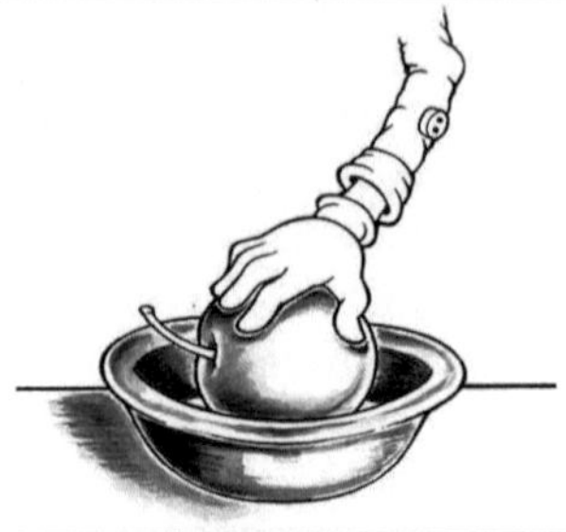	**FRUIT** Put fruit in bowl
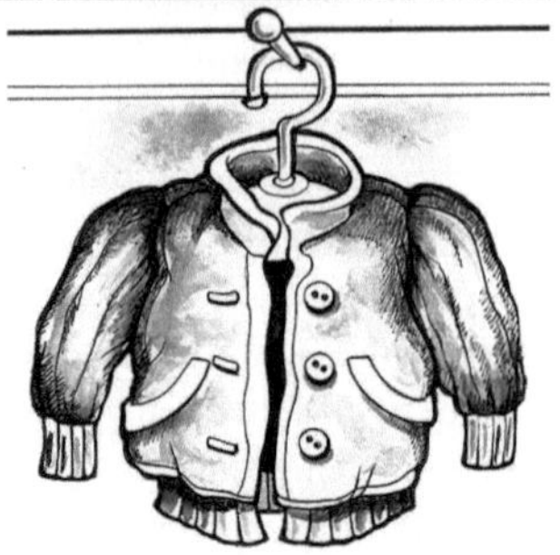	**JACKET** Hang up jacket
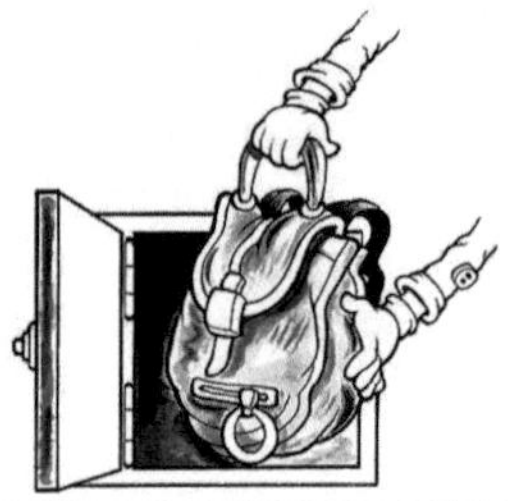	**BAG** Place bag in locker
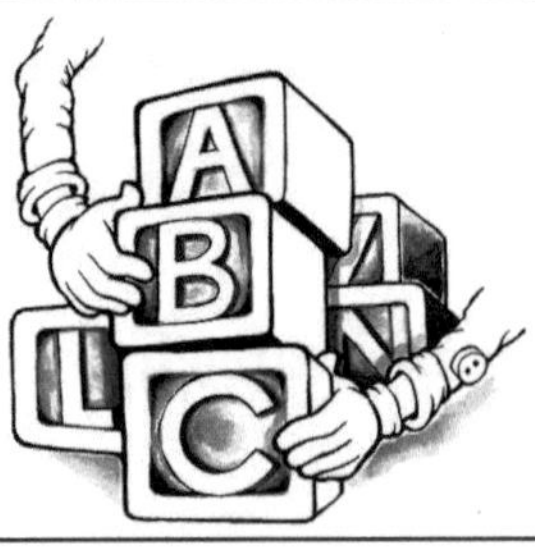	**PLAY** Find something to play with.

Fig. 5.2 Sequence of daily routine for preschoolers to enter the classroom

There is MRI evidence of a restorative benefit in terms of neural plasticity through cognitive training and in particular process-based interventions. The brain can be trained to develop new pathways and employ more efficient problem-solving practices particularly for individuals who have immature development or impairment of functioning.

Experience is a major stimulant of brain plasticity in animal species as diverse as insects and humans. It is now clear that experience produces multiple, dissociable changes in the brain including increases in dendritic length, increases (or decreases) in spine density, synapse formation, increased glial activity and altered metabolic activity. According to Kolb (1998), these anatomical changes are correlated with behavioural differences between subjects with and without the change.

There is evidence from Lumma et al. (2018) that changes in brain structure could be induced through the training of specific psychological abilities, for example, mindfulness-based attention, prosocial behaviour, perspective taking and multitasking performance. The authors investigated structural plasticity underlying training-induced change in the emotional self-concept after daily perspective-taking practice over 3 months. They found that change in emotional self-concept of the participants was associated with increased grey matter in the right medial prefrontal cortex extending into right dorsolateral prefrontal cortex.

In another study, the authors developed a cognitive training program to enhance the driving skills of the elderly and to measure the transfer effects and possible changes in neural plasticity. The program was designed to enhance processing speed, executive control, working memory, visual processing and divided attention which had all been suggested to have significant relevance to driving safety.

The authors involved three groups of elderly participants (60–75 years) and found that the experimental group which received the direct cognitive training showed significant improvements in processing speed and working memory as well as marginally significant improvement in executive function. This group displayed significant improvement in grey matter volume increases in the left orbito-frontal cortex.

In a study involving 46 elderly clients, the researchers found the strongest training effects following auditory perception training which resulted in long-term transfer to everyday problem solving and reasoning. This particular training group was also associated with changes in both the dorsal and ventral attention networks. In the ventral network, the authors found changed integrity of occipito-temporal white matter following the targeted training compared to each of the other training tasks. This change was associated with improved untrained everyday problem solving.

Kihwan et al. (2017) were able to demonstrate changes in cortical thickness and resting state connectivity of individuals at chronic stage of TBI following strategy-based reasoning training. The authors were of the view that theirs was the first MRI-based study to report brain plasticity as measured by both cortical thickness and resting state frontal connectivity following cognitive training.

Wintemute and colleagues (2012) discovered a metacognitive network within the brain that was engaged during the process of solving what they termed exception mathematical problems, those for which there was not a known technique. The metacognitive network included the angular gyrus, middle temporal gyrus and anterior prefrontal regions. They stated that the metacognitive network was mainly engaged by the need to modify the solution procedure and not by the difficulty of the problem.

Hardi Hossein and colleagues (2016) involved participants in a novel executive function task and provided them with real-time feedback about the level of brain activity or rhythm. Of the 20 healthy participants, 10 received real neurofeedback, and 10 received a sham feedback. Compared with the sham group, the neurofeedback group showed improved executive function performance, including improved performance on measures of working memory, after four sessions of a computerised training program. The neurofeedback group also showed significantly reduced training-related brain activity in the executive function network including right middle frontal and inferior frontal regions compared with the sham group.

The evidence from research studies supports the notion that cognitive rehabilitation training involving long-term changes in everyday functioning, whether this be in the realm of problem solving or other prosocial behaviour, can lead to changes in brain structure. It would follow that teaching clients to use a metacognitive strategy for problem solving that was eventually internalised and integrated into their everyday functioning was more than likely to result in a concomitant change in brain structure. For clients with TBI, ADHD, intellectual disability, CD, ASD and learning difficulty, this is a powerful message to send. It also raises the whole issue of brain plasticity and whether brain damage or immature development of the brain is permanent.

In a medico-legal situation, neuropsychologists are often asked to predict the long-term outcome of a client who may have sustained a significant traumatic brain injury. To what extent has the client's brain injury stabilised to the point where there would be no further improvement of function? I suggest, in view of the evidence for neural plasticity, this is a vexing question.

Take the example of my case study at the beginning of this book. My client sustained a significant traumatic brain injury and presented with significant dysexecutive function to the point where he failed his university course 2 years running following his injury. The dean of the college was in the process of terminating my client's enrolment at the university. At that point you would opine that he was not capable of completing his course and that he would drop out of university and have difficulty holding down a regular job and living independently. This would not be an unrealistic scenario.

However, I worked with him over a period of 12 months teaching him to use a metacognitive strategy which he embraced and internalised. The outcome was that he not only completed his course but also completed a PhD and then obtained a postdoctoral appointment overseas. You could not have predicted this outcome from his initial presentation!

I suggest my experience with this particular client and the many others I have worked with over the years have taught me that we need to be cautious about making long-term predictions regarding the effects of a traumatic brain injury.

References

Baron Levi, J. (1995). *Training adolescents with brain injuries to use a problem-solving plan.* Paper presented at the Second Pacific Rim Conference of the International Neuropsychological Society, Cairns, Australia.

Garcia, T., et al. (2016). Metacognition and executive functioning in elementary school. *Anales de Psicologia, 32*(2), 474–483.

Hardi Hossein, S. M., et al. (2016). Task-based neurofeedback training: a novel approach toward training executive functions. *NeuroImage, 134*, 153–159.

Kihwan, H., et al. (2017). Strategy-based reasoning training modulates cortical thickness and resting-state functional connectivity in adults with chronic traumatic brain injury. *Brain and Behaviour, 7*(5), 1–28.

Kolb, B., et al. (1998). Brain plasticity and behaviour. *Annual Review of Psychology, 49*, 43–64.

Lumma, A. L., et al. (2018). Change in emotional self-concept following socio-cognitive training relates to structural plasticity of the prefrontal cortex. *Brain and Behaviour, 8*(4), 1–15.

Lyons, K. E., & Ghetti, S. (2010). Metacognitive development in early childhood. New questions about old assumptions. In A. Elkides & P. Misaildi (Eds.), *Trends and prospects in metacognitive research* (pp. 259–278). New York: Springer.

Marulis, L. M., et al. (2016). Assessing metacognitive knowledge in 3–5 year olds: the development of a metacognitive knowledge interview. *Metacognition and Learning, 11*, 339–368.

Meichenbaum, D. (1977). *Cognitive-behavior modification: An integrative approach.* New York: Plenum.

Whitebread, D., Coltman, P., Pino Pasternak, D., Sangster, C., Grau, V., Bingham, S., Almeqdad, Q., & Demetriou, D. (2009). The development of two observational tools for assessing metacognition and self-regulated learning in young children. *Metacognition and Learning, 4*, 63–85.

Wintermute, S., et al. (2012). Brain networks supporting execution of mathematical skills versus acquisition of new mathematical competence. *PLoS, San Francisco, 7*(12), 1–19.

Ylvisaker, M., et al. (1994). A framework for cognitive intervention. In R. C. Savage & G. F. Wolcott (Eds.), *Educational dimensions of acquired brain injury*. Austin: Pro-Ed.

Chapter 6
Assessment

It is always advisable to conduct an assessment of adaptive behaviours such as executive functions, which measure metacognitive and behavioural/emotional functioning. In this way you can determine the strengths and weaknesses of the individual—build on their strengths and use these to compensate for their weaknesses.

Assessment of executive functions, in particular, can be complex because you are not just dealing with a unitary entity but a diverse range of skills and abilities. Because you are dealing with adaptive behaviour, I believe that an assessment should represent the environment in which the person is functioning. Neuropsychologists have been grappling with this issue for a long time, and many have come to the conclusion that ecological measures of executive function may assist in representing real-world behaviour of executive functioning.

Simon Crowe, an eminent Australian neuropsychologist made the point in a paper published in 2005 that most neuropsychological tests have not been empirically validated to predict the impact of impairment on activities of daily living or instrumental activities. According to Crowe, making the connection between the test result and the target behaviour is circumstantial at best.

Dr Silver (2000), in her seminal paper, stated that most neuropsychologists make the assumption that clinical tests have predictive power within the client's natural environment despite the fact that there is little research validating this assumption. Dr Silver advocated for the use of ecological measures in neuropsychology. She was of the view that to achieve ecological validity, a test must provide information that is relevant to the patient's functioning in daily life, not simply representative of a hypothetical construct or even a neurological syndrome. The central issue is the capacity of the assessment technique to answer questions about what to expect in the patient's everyday functioning and how to plan interventions and/or accommodations that will assist the individual in attaining optimal functioning.

Ylvisaker and Gioia (1998) point out that a client with TBI may perform poorly on an unfamiliar or unappealing test whereas functioning in a familiar routine may exceed expectations generated by the test results. Reviews of efficacy studies of

J. Baron Levi, *The Hairy Bikie and Other Metacognitive Strategies*,
https://doi.org/10.1007/978-3-030-46618-3_6

traditional neuropsychological tests have been critical of the capacity of these measures to assess functional, real-world outcomes and long-term maintenance of treatment gains. Similarly, Ylvisaker and colleagues (2003) concluded that the validity of contextualised or ecological measures had been found to be superior to standardised neuropsychological tests in the context of vocational planning after TBI. The authors also stated that apart from administering standard neuropsychological tests, contextualised observation is mandated by the frequent finding that people with TBI, particularly those with frontal lobe injury, often perform surprisingly better or worse in everyday contexts than can be predicted from standardised test performance.

A case in point was the example I gave in Chap. 2 of a client who tested poorly on standardised measures of executive functioning although was able to problem-solve an ingenious method of keeping birds away from his plants. He explained he had adapted a method he read on the Internet and applied it to his particular situation!

There are a number of assessments of executive functions that are based on ecological validity and measure real-world behaviour of the child or adolescent. The Behaviour Rating Inventory of Executive Function (BRIEF2), by Giola and colleagues (2015), is one such assessment that is often used as a measure of executive function. The BRIEF2 is a self-report inventory for parents and teachers for children and adolescents age 5–18 years and consists of eight theoretically and empirically derived clinical scales that assess behavioural manifestations of executive functioning. I have used the BRIEF over a number of years and have found it to be very useful in identifying specific aspects of executive functioning that I could work with in assisting a young person to be a more effective learner.

In 1991, while working for the NSW Department of Education with students with traumatic brain injuries, I spent some time searching for an appropriate measure of functional behaviours that I could apply to determine the extent of functional impairment of executive functioning. When I went into private practice, I developed my own measure based on the principles of ecological validity in that the assessment would contain a functional checklist of behaviours that represented the real world of the target students. The assessment was to be given to adults familiar with the students, such as their teachers or parents who were to rate each behaviour on a 4-point scale. The assessment contained statements that represented everyday real-world behaviours that related to executive functions in terms of metacognitive and emotional behaviours.

Functional Executive Scale (FES)
©Jeffrey Baron Levi 1994
Instructions: Please circle the number that relates to the frequency of occurrence of each behaviour, ensuring that you respond to every statement. Provide a brief comment where relevant.
Frequency of occurrence:
0 (never occurs), 1 (sometimes occurs), 2 (often occurs), 3 (always occur), Comment

1. Relates well with peers

0....1....2....3....

2. Maintains a positive attitude
   0....1....2....3....
3. Takes responsibility for self and own possessions
   0....1....2....3....
4. Appears confident in social situations
   0....1....2....3....
5. Is aware of other's feelings/viewpoint
   0....1....2....3....
6. Shows appropriate emotional response to peers
   0....1....2....3....
7. Shows appropriate emotional response to adults
   0....1....2....3....
8. Is able to learn from social experience
   0....1....2....3....
9. Is easily excitable
   0....1....2....3....
10. Obeys school/class rules
    0....1....2....3....
11. Accepts criticism
    0....1....2....3....
12. Responds to positive reinforcement/praise
    0....1....2....3....
13. Behaves badly toward peers
    0....1....2....3....
14. Is aware of own limitations/disability
    0....1....2....3....
15. Is able to make and maintain appropriate eye contact
    0....1....2....3....
16. Is able to position self at appropriate distance in conversation
    0....1....2....3....
17. Is able to control the amount of own talk
    0....1....2....3....
18. Is punctual to class
    0....1....2....3....
19. Is easily distracted by events around him/her
    0....1....2....3....
20. Remembers to bring appropriate materials to class
    0....1....2....3....
21. Asks for help if doesn't understand an activity/instruction
    0....1....2....3....
22. Works independently
    0....1....2....3....
23. Demonstrates appropriate organisation of self/materials

0....1....2....3....

24. Can concentrate and attend to a task for an expected period
0....1....2....3....
25. Is able to get started on a set activity without assistance
0....1....2....3....
26. Completes tasks within a reasonable time frame
0....1....2....3....
27. Shows pride in own work
0....1....2....3....
28. Copes with changes in routine
0....1....2....3....
29. Participates in class discussions
0....1....2....3....
30. Is able to follow and cope with topic changes
0....1....2....3....
31. Fatigues easily
0....1....2....3....
32. Remembers facts/information taught yesterday
0....1....2....3....
33. Is able to follow all steps of a particular activity
0....1....2....3....
34. Is able to respond to verbal instructions within an appropriate time frame
0....1....2....3....
35. Can make inferences and draw conclusions
0....1....2....3....
36. Is able to retell events/story
0....1....2....3....
37. Anticipates consequences/thinks ahead
0....1....2....3....
38. Is able to "pick up" on new information
0....1....2....3....
39. Demonstrates understanding of written instructions
0....1....2....3....
40. Has adequate planning skills—can logically set out an essay
0....1....2....3....
41. Shows awareness when doesn't understand an activity/task
0....1....2....3....
42. Remembers an instruction and follows through without forgetting
0....1....2....3....
43. Demonstrates adequate problem-solving skills
0....1....2....3....
44. Behaves badly toward authority figures
0....1....2....3....

Functional Executive Scale (FES)
List of item numbers that relate to each of the subscales

Metacognitives	**Behavioural/emotional**
3	
	1
10	**2**
13	**4**
17	**5**
18	**6**
19*	**7**
20	**8**
21	**9***
22	**11**
23	**12**
24	
26	**14**
28	**15**
29	**16**
30	**25**
32	**27**
33	**31***
34	**44**
35	
36	
37	
38	
39	
40	
41	
42	
43	
N = 27	**N = 17**

***Negative item-scoring to be reversed**

Once the checklist has been scored, it is then possible to construct a profile of strengths and weaknesses. Table 6.1 is an example of a secondary student's profile which was constructed from the result of the behaviour checklist.

Table 6.1 Naomi's plan from the results of the FES

Naomi		
Year 9 high school:		
Domains	Strengths	Weaknesses
Emotional	Relates well to peers	
	Has a positive attitude	
	Responds to praise	
Metacognitive	Average to high average working memory	Reduced self-monitoring
		Concentration problematic
		Poor organisation
		Difficulty getting started.
		Poor problem-solving
		Poor inferential skills

Naomi's Profile Based on the FES

Naomi, a secondary school student, was experiencing difficulty with her schoolwork. She had been involved in a motor vehicle accident some years earlier and had suffered a moderate traumatic brain injury. She received additional support throughout her primary school grades although received no support in secondary school because she moved to the private sector and information about her earlier difficulties was not communicated to her new school. She was referred for an assessment.

Rehabilitation Plan Based on Test Results

A cognitive rehabilitation plan for Naomi was then developed on the basis of the test profile. It was apparent that Naomi was experiencing difficulty with executive functioning, particularly in organising her time, initiating school work, becoming distracted in the classroom and slow to complete set work.

I sat down with Naomi and her teacher and explained the test results and the profile. I asked Naomi to go through the process of how she worked in the classroom to complete set work, from the moment she was given the work to her approach to working on the problem. Her response confirmed the results of the assessment. However, it was also the case that if she became stuck on a particular part or problem, she tended not to ask for help or assistance. Together we worked out a plan that would assist Naomi to overcome some of these problems with her learning.

Naomi's Plan

Following the functional assessment and discussions with Naomi, we arrived at some learning and executive function issues that needed to be addressed.

Fig. 6.1 Problem Solving Plan

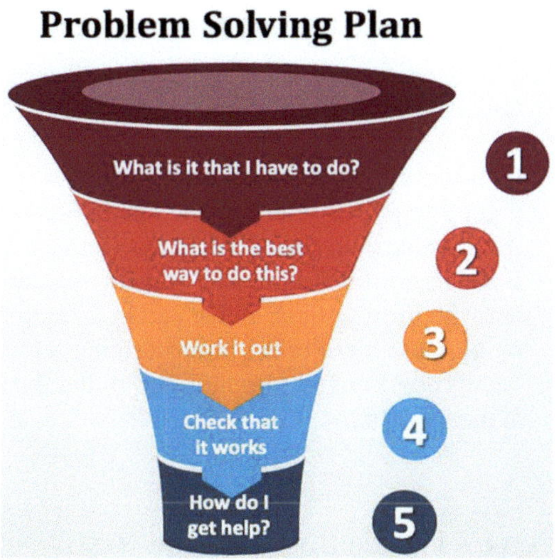

The following is the plan that was developed in collaboration with Naomi and her teacher (Fig. 6.1):

What is it that I have to do?
What is the important information that is provided?
Highlight the information so that I will remember it.
Read and reread.
What does the problem/question ask me to do?
Do I understand what the question is about?

What is the best way to do it?
How can I work out the problem?
What strategies can I use?
Brainstorm some ideas. Think of as many ideas as you can.
Write them down. Figure out which ones may work.
Can you break the problem into smaller parts?

How do I get help?
If I can't work it out then who can help me?
Ask the teacher or another student to help.

Do it!
I can now work out the problem. Keep working on it until it is finished.
Don't get distracted!

Check that it works
Have I answered all of the questions?
Does my answer make sense?
Check over how I worked it out.
Ask the teacher to check your work.

The Plan was written on a card for Naomi to keep on her desk.

The instructions for the teacher were as follows:

- Encourage Naomi to follow the Plan.
- If you see her working on the Plan, give her positive attention.
- If she appears to be stuck, or distracted or not working, then ask her: Where are you up to on the Plan? Encourage her to work through the steps. What do you think the next step should be? Don't give her the answer.
- If she has difficulty moving forward at a particular step in the Plan, then prompt her with the questions at that particular step. You may need to assist her in developing more ideas in the brainstorming section. Try to ask "how" or "where" or "why" questions to stimulate her to find the answers in order to get her to arrive at the solution.

Peter's Profile Based on the Results of the FES

Peter, a Year 5 student, was referred because of behavioural and learning difficulties. He had been diagnosed with ADHD several years earlier and had been trialled on medication although currently drug free. His teacher was concerned about his behaviour in the classroom as he was disrupting the other students and highly distractible in the classroom.

His profile on the FES is detailed in Table 6.2.

I developed a rehabilitation plan for Peter and his teacher based on the results of the FES.

I had earlier asked his teacher to take observational notes on when Peter's behaviour became an issue. I wanted her to identify what were the apparent triggers for Peter's behaviour and in doing so to determine the general antecedents that precipitated his behavioural problems in the classroom and then her response to his behaviour. This approach is the ABC of behavioural intervention: Antecedents-Behaviour-Consequences. We determined that she may have been

Table 6.2 Peter's profile from the results of the FES

Peter		
Year 5 primary school:		
Domains	Strengths	Weaknesses
Emotional/ behavioural		Difficulty accepting criticism
		Difficulty relating to others
		Poorly behaved and difficulty following school and class rules
Metacognitive		Reduced self-monitoring
		Concentration problematic
		Poor organisation
		Poor problem-solving

rewarding a lot of his behaviour unnecessarily by giving him attention when he was acting inappropriately. We also determined that Peter acted out when he was given work that he found too challenging and then his behaviour escalated when his teacher admonished him.

So, we had a number of issues that we needed to work on: providing Peter with work at his level, teaching him to control his behaviour and for his teacher to take more notice of him when he was acting appropriately rather than inappropriately. Of course, if Peter's behaviour was so bad that he was totally out of control, his teacher needed to intervene.

I have included Peter's rehabilitation plan in Chap. 11, Behaviour Management.

References

Crowe, S. (2005). The parallel universe: Does neuropsychological assessment tell us anything about the real world? *Australian Psychological Society: Inpsych June 2005.*

Gioia, G. A., Isquith, P. K., Guy, S. C., & Kenworthy, L. (2015). *Behavior rating inventory of executive function, second edition (BRIEF2).* Odessa, Florida: Psychological Assessment Resources.

Silver, C. H. (2000). Ecological validity of neuropsychological assessment in childhood traumatic brain injury. *Journal of Head Trauma Rehabilitation, 15*(4), 973–988. (p 974).

Ylvisaker, M., & Gioia, G. A. (1998). Cognitive assessment. In M. Ylvisaker (Ed.), *Traumatic brain injury rehabilitation: Children and adolescents* (2nd ed., pp. 159–179). Boston: Butterworth-Heinmann.

Yvlisaker, M., et al. (2003). Rehabilitation of children and adults with cognitive-communication disorders after brain injury: Ad hoc committee on interprofessional. *ASHA's Annual Supplement, 8*(7), 59–72.

Chapter 7
The Hairy Bikie

The Hairy Bikie Problem Solver (HBMPC) was one example of a generic Problem Solving Plan that I developed as a process that could be applied across any content area. I used it with students in the classroom as a structured approach to working through problems. I had the HBMPC steps printed on a small card which the students kept on their desks for easy reference. Teacher's aides also prompted the students to use the approach with the emphasis on training the student to independently apply the strategies. Prompting was in regard to the processes rather than the content. So, the prompts may be "Where are you up to with your plan?", "What is the next step?" and "Do you know how to work it out?" rather than giving the student the answers. It was always about teaching the students the processes so that they would internalise them and become independent learners. The processes were in fact a type of frontal lobe prosthesis!

The four components of the HBMPC model as with all of the Problem Solving Plans I developed with students and adults are detailed in Table 7.1.

The **alerting** function is alerting the person to what they need to do, recognising that there is an issue they need to work on or attending to or stopping what they are doing and taking notice as in the case of acting or behaving inappropriately at the time. It can be about putting up a STOP sign or devising a signal which the teacher or therapist works out in conjunction with the student or client to alert them to take notice.

The **recalling/acting** function is reminding the person of the techniques or strategies that they have learned to solve the problem or the issue at hand. It is then time to put those strategies or skills into action and do it! Do you remember what you need to do? Tell me how you are going to solve this problem or work this out?

The **monitoring/checking** function involves keeping in working memory the goal you are attempting to achieve and then working on the issue without being distracted until the goal is achieved or the work completed. At every step you need to keep monitoring what you are working on to ensure you are using all of the critical information and answering the question. In the case of behaviour management, for example, monitoring may involve monitoring your level of stress or tension and

J. Baron Levi, *The Hairy Bikie and Other Metacognitive Strategies*,
https://doi.org/10.1007/978-3-030-46618-3_7

Table 7.1 Four components of a metacognitive strategy

Alerting	Take notice. Focus!	STOP! LISTEN!	
Recalling/ acting	You know what to do	You have learned the skills	Do it!
Monitoring/ checking		Work on it! Put the skills into action!	Keep checking/working on it!
Verifying	Is it working?	Check you have completed the task. Did you follow the instructions?	Did you use all of the given information?

Table 7.2 Example of a self-monitoring proforma

Behaviour	Sometimes	Often	Always
I was able to complete all of the work in class			
I remembered what I had to do			
I came to class with homework completed			
I was able to use the Hairy Bikie			

focus on calming yourself during the process of removing yourself from an anger-producing situation. One technique I have often used is to draw up a monitoring proforma and ask the client to chart their progress or success along the way. This technique can be a powerful method for behaviour change when you are asked to record your behaviour or success at using a particular strategy (Table 7.2).

The **verifying** function is checking that you have actually achieved the goal you set out to achieve or completed the task using all of the information that you were given. Did you follow all of the instructions using all of the important information? You need to ask yourself: "When I refer back to the question or the task, does my response make sense?"

The steps above are the essential components of a metacognitive strategy. I like to add a fifth component which is to reward or congratulate yourself for successfully solving the problem or putting the skills into action to get a positive outcome.

The reward function would therefore be an optional step in the process.

To make it easy to remember, particularly for younger students, I made up the following mnemonic for the HBMPC problem-solver:

Hairy Bikie Munches Pop Corn (HBMPC) (Highlight, Brainstorm, Map, Process, Check)

Map

I'll explain in detail what each of the steps in the process involves. But I want to pay particular attention to the notion of mapping. What is a MAP? There are a number of variations of mapping including concept mapping, mind mapping and even scaffolding which is a type of visual representation. All have been used in education and rehabilitation and represent a way of visually representing a concept or idea so that it can then be expanded or built and used to generate additional ideas or to problem-solve. From my experience, clients who have problematic working memory do benefit from a visual representation of the information at hand. They can actually "see" what it is that they are working on, and this often prompts them to generate more ideas to problem-solve.

The idea of a "map" may simply involve drawing the concept or making a diagram of the information so that it can be visually represented. Often seeing the information set out visually can be a prompt to working out the answer. And given that the clients we are assisting often have difficulty with working memory, then a visual representation of the information can often greatly assist in working through the problem.

Figure 7.1 is an example of a mind map that I developed in conjunction with a female client who was completing her last year of school and considering her career options. We worked through each of her choices and looked at the merits of each, what kind of training would be required and how she would be able to find work in her chosen field. The mind map then became a visual plan for carrying out an action, and by representing it visually, it became a road map for action. Once we had the basic ideas down on paper, we then added further points to elaborate on particular aspects of the plan. The map became dynamic, a living plan. One of the issues she raised was whether she would be accepted as a female motor mechanic, so we used the map as a means of exploring that issue.

So, mind maps are a way of visually representing your ideas. They allow you to let your ideas and associations flow freely. They are a method of combining brainstorming, predicting outcomes, discovering relationships and planning. For this reason they are a useful technique for clients who are experiencing difficulty in putting their ideas on paper or initiating a set task. They can be the first step in the planning process.

It is also a useful technique for clients who have difficulty processing a lot of information, or those who have problematic verbal memory. To this end I have found mind maps to be particularly effective with clients with dysexecutive function or significant learning difficulties. For these clients mind maps are a method of visually organising and visually planning information from which they can then begin to problem-solve.

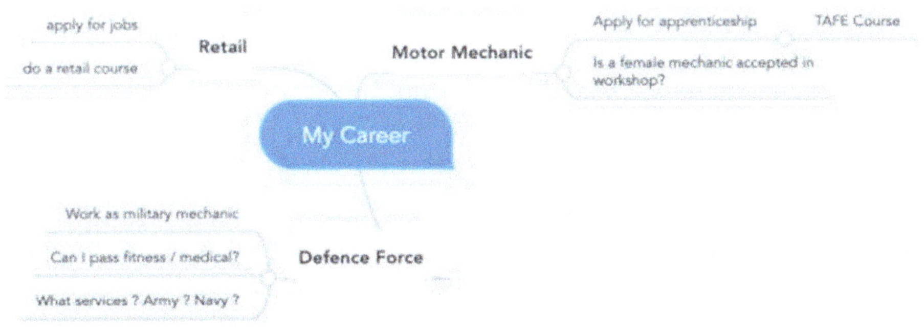

Fig. 7.1 My Career Options Mind Map

Hairy Bikie Munches Pop Corn

Step 1: WHAT DO YOU HAVE TO DO?
What are you asked to do?
What is the important information you have been given?
HIGHLIGHT the important information.
Do you understand what you have to do?
Not sure who can you ask for help?
Who did you ask?

Step 2: HOW ARE YOU GOING TO DO IT? BRAINSTORM/BREAK IT DOWN.
Brainstorm some ideas.
Think of as many ideas as you can—write them down. Figure out which ones might work.
Break the problem down into smaller steps/parts/chunks. Do each step separately.
Make a list including materials or equipment you will need.

Step 3: MAP
Draw a mind map setting out how you would work through the problem.
Make sure you work it out in the right order.
What is the first thing you would do?
What is the next thing?
Not sure who can you ask for help?
Who did you ask?

Step 4: DO IT! PROCESS
Keep working out the problem until it is finished.
Stay focused!
Don't get distracted!
Remember what you are doing.
Keep checking back with the important information you wrote down.
Are you stuck?
Ask for help.
Who did you ask?
Congratulate yourself!

Step 5: CHECK IT
Check that you carried out all of the steps.
Go back and look at the information you were given.
Did you do it in the right order?
Did you use the right materials/tools/equipment?
Does your answer make sense?
Ask someone to check your work.
Who did you ask?

Excellent work!
Problem-Solving Using the Hairy Bikie Strategy (Fig. 7.2)

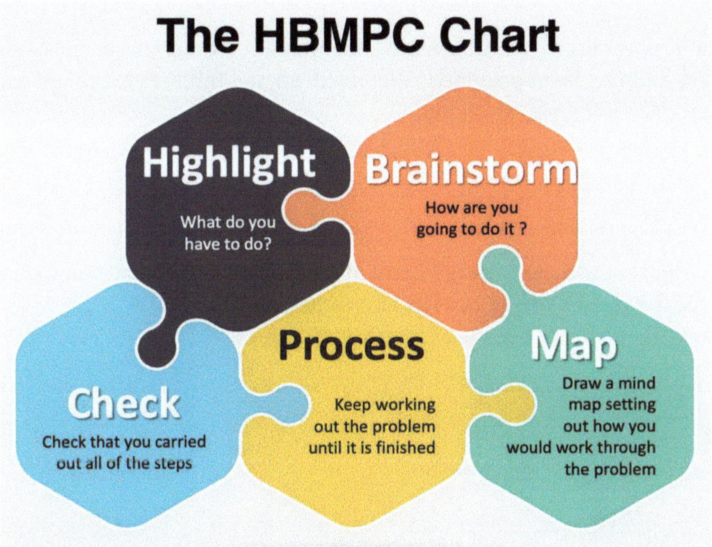

Fig. 7.2 The HBMPC Chart

Problem One:
Four members of a junior soccer team, David, Sean, Kevin and Kieran, are sitting around a table after a soccer match. They are drinking Solo, Pepsi, lemonade and mineral water. In their last soccer match, one of them scored 2 goals, one scored 1 goal, a third was given a yellow card and a fourth was given a red card. ***Find which player scored 2 goals and which one was drinking Solo.***

1. David does not drink mineral water.
2. Sean invites the player sitting next to him to have a Pepsi.
3. The player who scored 1 goal is opposite the one who was given a yellow card.
4. The player who scored 2 goals is sitting to the left of the Pepsi drinker.
5. Kevin is sitting opposite the player who scored 2 goals.
6. The player who was given a red card is drinking mineral water.
7. Kieran thanks Sean for the drink.
8. The player who was given a yellow card was drinking Solo.

Highlight
I have highlighted the question that needs to be answered. We need to keep this in focus.

Brainstorm/Break it Down
How are we going to work out the answer? We could draw a diagram setting out where each player may be sitting. We could go through the 7 points and try to logically work it out using that information.

Map

Let's draw a diagram of where each of the players would be seated based on the information that has been provided. We can draw the table and arrange each of the players based on what we do know.

Process

Do it!

Step 1:

Where are the four players sitting? Draw the table and see if you can locate them. Sean invites the player sitting next to him to have a Pepsi.
So we know the Pepsi drinker is either side of Sean.

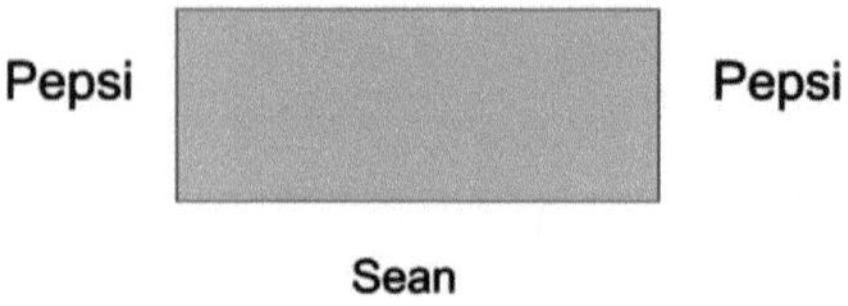

Step 2:

Kieran thanks Sean for the drink. So, we know that Kieran is the Pepsi drinker. He could be sitting either side of Sean.

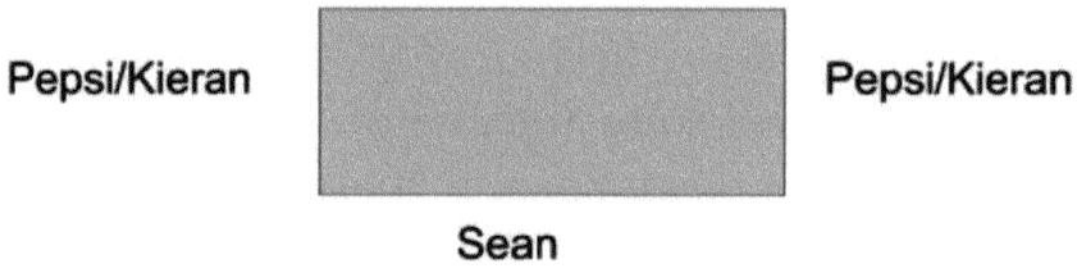

Step 3:

The player who scored 2 goals is sitting to the left of the Pepsi drinker. So we know that the player who scored 2 goals could be Sean, David or Kevin.

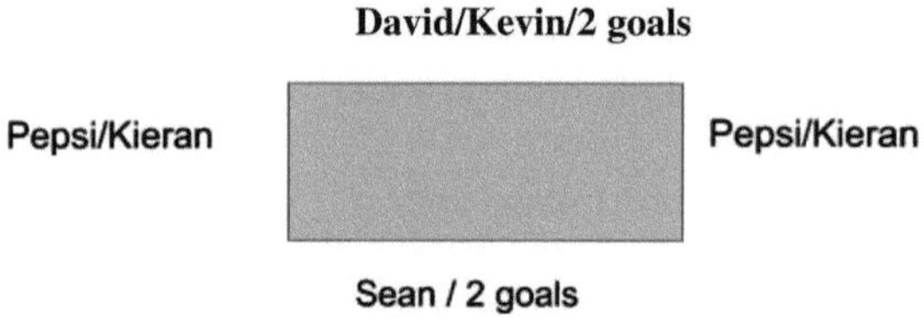

Step 4:

Kevin is sitting opposite the player who scored 2 goals.

So, we now know that Kevin did not score the 2 goals. We also know now that if Kevin is seated opposite the player who scored 2 goals, then it must be Sean who scored the 2 goals.

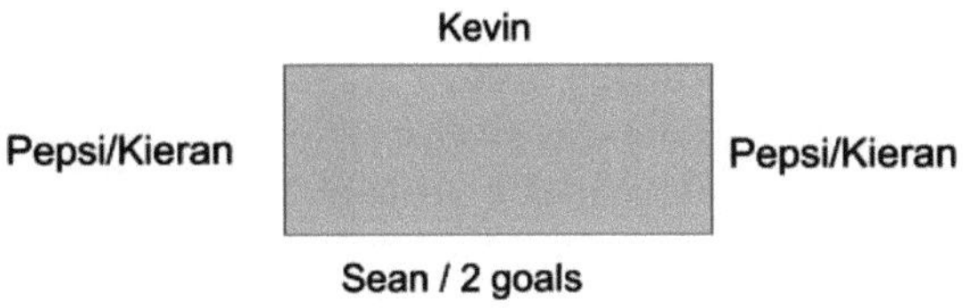

Step 5:

The player who scored 1 goal is opposite the one who was given a yellow card. So we know that either David or Kieran scored 1 goal or was given a yellow card.

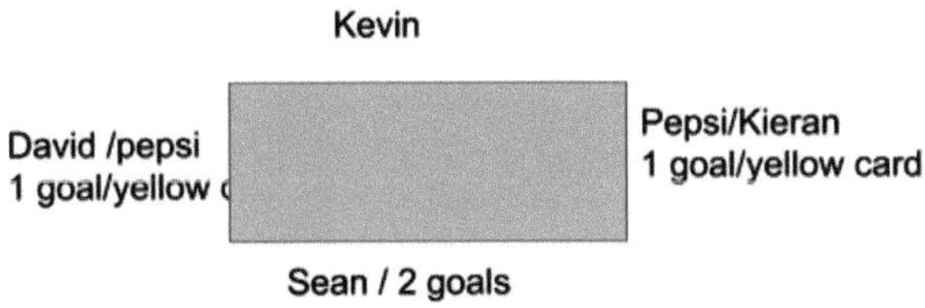

Step 6:

David does not drink mineral water.

So we know that David drinks either lemonade or Solo and either Kevin or Sean must drink mineral water.

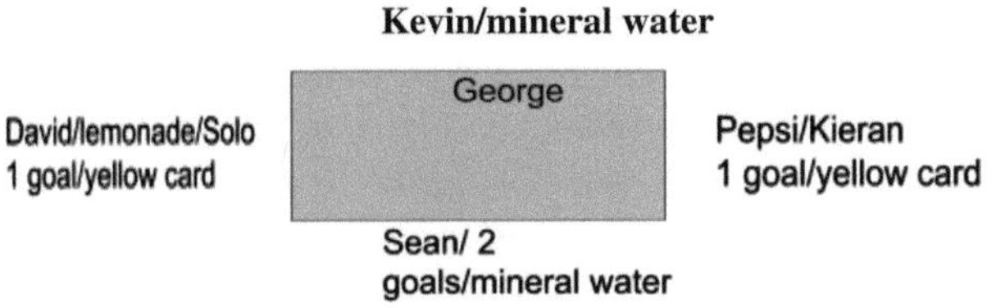

Step 7:

The player who was given a red card is drinking mineral water.

So now we know that Kevin was given a red card as we have already established he was drinking mineral water.

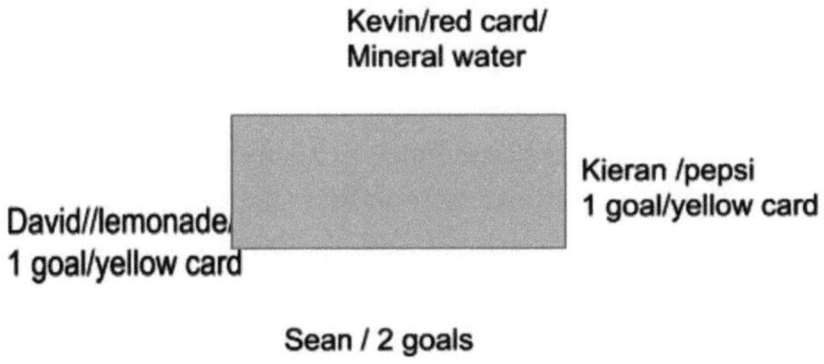

Step 8:

The player who was given a yellow card was drinking Solo.

So, now we know that David was drinking Solo and was given a yellow card, Kieran scored 1 goal and was drinking Pepsi, Sean scored 2 goals and was drinking lemonade, and Kevin was drinking mineral water and given a red card.

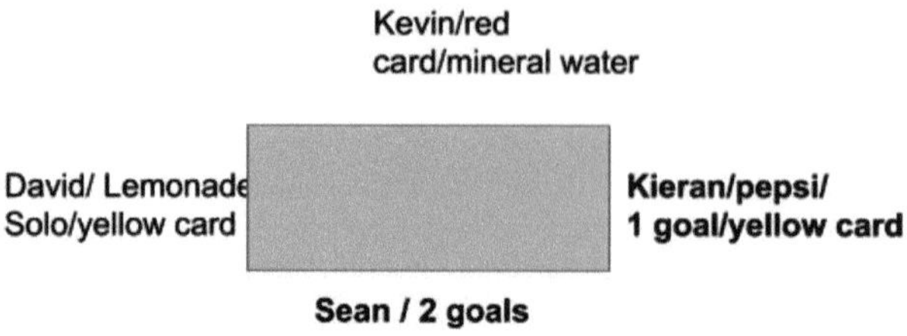

Answer:

We can now answer the question: *Find which player scored 2 goals and which one was drinking Solo.* **Sean scored the 2 goals, and David was drinking Solo.**

Check

Go through the 8 points again and check that you have inserted the correct information.

Problem Two:

It's 5 pm and you are expected for an important meeting in Melbourne at 9 am the next morning. There are two flights available. One is a flight that leaves at 9 pm and arrives in Melbourne at 7:30 am the next day. The other flight departs at 10 pm and arrives in Melbourne at 8.30 am the next day. When you arrive in Melbourne, you will need to wait 20 minutes for your luggage, and it will take 30 minutes by Uber to get to your meeting. ***Which flight will you take, and will you have time to buy breakfast before the meeting?***

Step 1: Highlight the question

It is highlighted so that you don't forget.

Step 2: Brainstorm/break it down

You need to break the problem down by examining each step. The second step, "B", brainstorm/break it down. We'll start from the time the planes land in Melbourne and then work forward on a timeline toward the meeting time to see which flight would work the best.

Step 3: Map

Let's draw a timeline starting from the time the plane lands in Melbourne and working forward toward the 9 am meeting time to see which flight would work.

Early Flight

7:30 am	7:50 am	8:20 am	9 am
Plane arrives Melbourne	**Pick up bags**	**Catch Uber**	**Meeting**

Later Flight

8:30 am	8:50 am	9:20 am	9 am
Plane arrives Melbourne	**Pick up bags**	**Catch Uber**	**Meeting**

Step 4: Process

You can immediately see that the later flight arrives in Melbourne at 8:30 am which is already too late because by the time you wait 20 minutes for the baggage and then the 30-minute Uber ride, it is already after 9 am, so you would miss the 9 am appointment.

The answer is that you catch the earlier flight and you arrive at 8:20 am which is in time to have breakfast before the 9 am meeting.

Step 5: Check

Go back and check the timeline again and make sure you have entered the correct times.

Problem Three:

Assuming that four of these dates are correct, which one is wrong:

1. *Monday, 10 January 1804*
2. *Monday, 24 January 1804*
3. *Monday, 14 February 1804*
4. *Monday, 7 March 1804*
5. *Monday, 3 April 1804*

The first thing we should do is **highlight** the question: I have highlighted it in red. So we know we are looking for the one wrong date.

We need to **brainstorm** or break it down. How are we going to work out the answer? What do we know? They are all in the same year, all within a few months of each other and all fall on a Monday. Let's start with the first date and count on from there.

Can we draw a timeline or **map** the date? Yes we can! We can log each Monday from 10 January.

10 Jan, 17 Jan, 24 Jan, 31 Jan, 7 Feb, 14 Feb, 21 Feb, 28 Feb

We stop here because we now need to consider is this a leap year? What do you think? Leap years occur every 4 years. How do we tell if it is a leap year? If the year can be evenly divided by 4, then it is a leap year.

1804 can be evenly divided by 4, so it IS a leap year which means we go to February 29.

Returning to our timeline:

10 Jan, 17 Jan, 24 Jan, 31 Jan, 7 Feb, 14 Feb, 21 Feb, 28 Feb, 6 March, 13 March, 20 March, 27 March, 3 April, 10 April

So now we **process** the information we have placed on our timeline.

We can now compare our dates on the timeline with the information we have been given and check which ones we have listed and which is the wrong date. You can see from the given dates which are highlighted above that 7 March 1804 is the wrong date as it should be 6 March 1804. All of the other dates are on our timelines.

Let's **check** our answer. Did you answer correctly? You should go over the question to make sure you answered the question and that you used all of the information that was given. Then you should check that the timeline is correct. If all works out, then congratulations!

YOU DID IT!

Problem Four:

You and three friends are planning a driving holiday from Sydney to Brisbane, stopping overnight at two locations—Taree and Southport. You want to go during the Christmas holidays, leaving Sydney on 18 December. You want to stay 2 nights in each town in which you stop and then 3 nights in Brisbane. You want to rent a car to drive to Brisbane, and then you all want to fly home from Brisbane to Sydney. How would you go about planning this holiday?

Highlight

What is the important information?

- When you want to leave Sydney. When you leave Brisbane.
- Four people travelling.
- Rent a car from Sydney to Brisbane.
- Stay 2 nights each at Taree and Southport and 3 in Brisbane.
- Leave rental car in Brisbane and then fly home to Sydney.

Brainstorm/Break it down

How are we going to plan this trip? What do we need to do first? We should break down the various components of the trip and then brainstorm each component.

1. Book 2 nights Taree and Southport and 3 nights Brisbane. Hotel or Airbnb? How many rooms? How do we find accommodation? Where do we want to stay in each town/city?
2. Book return airfare Brisbane to Sydney. What airline do we use? When do we leave?
3. Arrange rental car. Who do we use? Who will be the designated driver? What type of car will we need for four people and luggage? Do we need the car in Brisbane or do we drop it off when we arrive? How will we get around in Brisbane for the 3 days?

4. How will we pay?
5. What do we pack for the trip? We need to be under 20 kg per suitcase for the flight home.

Map

We need to map out the list of activities needed to prepare for this trip. We should do this in sequence and make a list, in order, detailing what needs to be done:

Accommodation: Draw a timeline

Leave Sydney in 18 December.
Early: arrive Taree later that day.
Stay overnight in 18 and 19 December.
Leave for Southport in 20 December.
Arrive Southport later that day.
Overnight Southport in 20 and 21 December.
Leave for Brisbane in 22 December; arrive later that day.
Overnight Brisbane in 22, 23 and 24 December and leave in 25 December. Where do we want to stay in Brisbane?

Draw a mind map with the following in the centre:

Car hire: Research companies on the Internet (van/large car). Can we pick up Sydney and drop off Brisbane?
Airfare: Google airfares one-way Brisbane to Sydney. Economy class. How much luggage can we take? Departure and arrival times? How do we get to and from the airports?
Preparation: What do we need to pack? How many suitcases? No more than 20 kg in weight (Fig. 7.3).

Process

You should now have a detailed plan of what you need to do to organise this trip.

Accommodation: Go on Internet sites and check out accommodation in Taree, Southport and Brisbane. Compare prices and availability for hotel or an apartment on Airbnb. Compare prices and dates. Book!
Airline: Book return airfare Brisbane to Sydney 25 December. Make sure booked luggage of 20 kg is included. Allow enough time to get to the airport.
Car hire: Book large car or van to accommodate four people and luggage leaving Sydney in 18 December and drop off Brisbane.
Preparation: Pack sufficient clothes for 8 days, including additional clothes you may want to wear during the evening—one suitcase per person plus hand luggage for the plane.

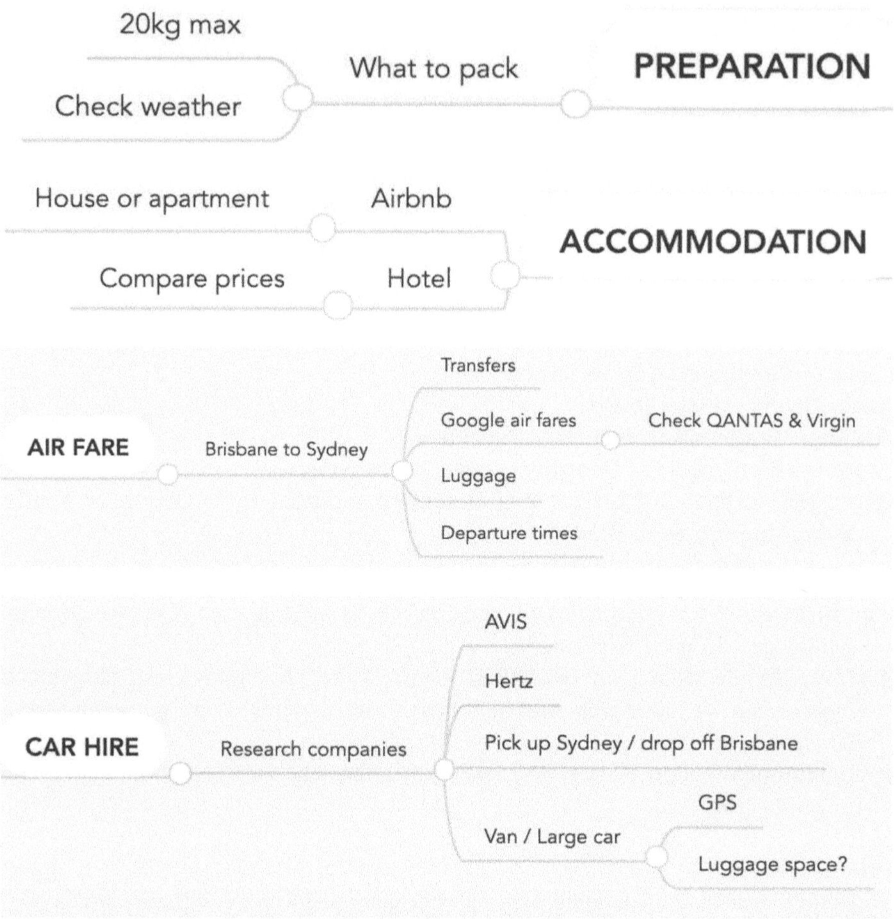

Fig. 7.3 Mind Map of Holiday Planning

Chapter 8
More Case Studies and Strategies

Developing an Individual Approach to Problem Solving

Often, when I am working with students and we identify there is an issue, we work together to find the words that they can use and understand in a sequence of steps to overcome that problem. The problem has often been identified by a third party such as a teacher or parent who may tell me the student has a problem staying on task or remembering what it is they have to do or it may be they present with challenging behaviours. These problems may occur in the classroom, at home or out in the community.

So, for example, I may ask the student to tell me in their own words what happens when they are doing a task and become distracted. Are they aware they go off-task? What are the distractors? Do they forget what they were doing? Do they become distracted in all situations?

I will then go back to the third party and verify the information provided by the student. Is this what the teacher/parent is also observing?

We then build up a picture that can lead to a possible solution.

Together with the third person and the student, we begin to identify steps in a process that will teach the student how to avoid distractions and stay on task to complete an activity. In effect we are sequencing the steps the student needs to work through to overcome the identified issue of concern.

I will go through the same process with challenging behaviours or problematic memory. In these particular cases, the Hairy Bikie strategy may not be appropriate as we are not solving a "problem" per se but working toward assisting the student to overcome or compensate for a particular deficit that is causing a problem for them or the people they are working with. The "problem" as such is with the person, and we are searching for a solution that will assist them to be a better learner and a better participant.

J. Baron Levi, *The Hairy Bikie and Other Metacognitive Strategies*,
https://doi.org/10.1007/978-3-030-46618-3_8

Staying on Task

Here is one example that I worked through with a student who was experiencing issues in staying on task to complete an activity.

Go through a dialogue with the student and teacher.

STOP!
WHAT DO YOU HAVE TO DO?
FOCUS!
DO IT!

These steps were printed on a card which was kept in front of the student as a reference point. In the classroom the teacher or parent, who was involved in developing the steps with the student, would take notice of the student when they were on task and not distracted, thereby "catching them out being good" and giving positive attention. If the teacher or parent became aware that the student was off-task, then they would simply say, "Stop! Where are you up to?", and encourage the student to follow the steps. Often we developed little signals that the teacher could use in an unobtrusive way so that they were not embarrassed by the rest of the class. The teacher may say "Class Listen!" and then make eye contact with the targeted student. The student knows the teacher is referring to him or her, but it is done in a way that does not draw particular attention to that student.

It is important that there is no negative attention given to the student, only a prompt of where they were up to in their plan.

Daniel

Injuries

Daniel, age 14 years, was hit by a car while riding his bicycle. He sustained a severe traumatic brain injury with bleeding on the brain and brain swelling. CT scans revealed a right base of skull fracture and left parietal bone fracture. There were bilateral contusions of the frontal lobes.

Concerns Following Return to School

Assessment on the FES and observations of Daniel's behaviour in the classroom revealed that the majority of Daniel's teachers had indicated failure to follow school and class rules, impulsive behaviour and failure to monitor his behaviour and initiate tasks were all of major concern. Daniel's profile from the FES was detailed in Table 8.1.

Table 8.1 Daniel's profile from the results of the FES

Executive Function Domain	Strengths	Weaknesses
Emotional/behavioural		Verbally and physically aggressive
		Impulsive behaviour
		Does not obey class rules
Metacognitive	Average general ability	Difficulty completing activities
	Average memory skills	Poor planning skills
		Poor concentration
		Does not work independently

Management Programme

There were two aspects to a management plan which would enable Daniel to be maintained in mainstream education. The first was recommended teaching strategies which had proven effective when teaching students with traumatic brain injuries. The second aspect to Daniel's intervention program was the direct teaching of strategies which would enable Daniel to take more control of his learning as well as the provision of support to assist him to implement these strategies. The second aspect involved the development of a Problem Solving Plan which would be taught in a one-on-one situation and then reinforced in the classroom by his teacher.

The development of the management programme was based on the principle that if Daniel was staying on task, checking what it was that he had to do and working on set tasks, then this had to be incompatible with breaking class rules! The assumption was that Daniel's impulsive behaviour and inability to consider the consequences of his actions were the result of dysexecutive function which resulted in poor planning and problem-solving skills. By providing Daniel with the structure for problem-solving and teaching him planning skills, then there was every likelihood Daniel would take control of his behaviour.

Problem Solving Plan

I sat down with Daniel and talked about his teacher's concerns and the behaviours that they had identified. I asked him whether he agreed with these observations and whether that was something that he wanted to work on. I suggested that if he could take control of these behaviours, then his time in school would be more enjoyable and he would get his teacher "off his back" as it were. He would also learn more and do well in school as he clearly had the ability to do so.

Together we identified the specific behaviours that we needed to work on in the classroom.

We chose three that appeared to be of most concern to his teachers.

I talked about Problem Solving Plans that had worked for other children who were having similar problems to Daniel. I explained in simple terms what a

Problem Solving Plan looked like. It was a step-by-step method that helped you work through problems, stay on task and follow the class rules. It had worked for many children and helped them to gain control of their learning.

Daniel agreed to work with me, and together with his teachers, we worked out a Problem Solving Plan.

The Plan was as follows:

Step 1: STOP!

Teachers would alert Daniel that he was off-task, distracted and not working on set tasks. We developed a signal between his teachers and Daniel so that Daniel was not always the negative focus of the classroom. The teachers would say "Class Listen!" and gain eye contact with Daniel. This was his signal that he was off-task.

Step 2: WHAT DO I NEED TO DO?

Teachers would approach Daniel and check that he knows what he has to do. He tells the teacher in his own words what he is working on and where he is up to.

Step 3: HOW AM I GOING TO DO IT?

Teachers ask Daniel how he is going to complete the task? Does he know what to do to work out the problem? What is the best way to do it? Can he break the problem down into smaller chunks?

Step 4: DO IT!

I know what to do! Get on with it and work out the problem. Keep working and don't get distracted.

Step 5: DO I NEED TO ASK FOR HELP?

If I get stuck at any time, I can ask the teacher to help me.

Step 6: HAVE I ANSWERED THE QUESTION?

Check that my answer makes sense. Look at the question again and make sure that I have used all of the information to answer the question. Check over how I worked it out.

Daniel was taught to follow these steps when working on particular problems in the classroom. In the beginning it would take a number of sessions of rehearsing the steps and asking Daniel to check that he knew what each step meant and that he was able to follow the Plan.

I used real situations in Mathematics and English to begin with to teach him to generalise the Plan to other subject areas. The Plan was printed on stick-on labels which Daniel placed at the back of each of his writing books for easy reference. I also asked Daniel to self-monitor how well he was able to initiate and complete activities using the Plan. I developed a self-monitoring chart for him to complete.

As Daniel was motivated to improve his learning, he did eventually internalise the steps and use them to effect. We made some minor adjustments to the program, based on teacher observations and the results of Daniel's self-monitoring charts as well as feedback from his parents.

In addition to the Problem Solving Plan, I also made some recommendations regarding teaching strategies for Daniel. Given that he had difficulty with planning, problem solving and learning in general, I suggested that the following strategies would provide the necessary processing simplifications that he was unable to apply himself. These strategies would work in tandem with the Problem Solving Plan. I was of the view that the teaching strategies would assist other students in the classroom who were also having difficulty with their learning.

Teaching Strategies

- Make the aim of the lesson clear at the beginning. Summarise at the end.
- Link new work to previous work (go through Daniel's book and show him what leads on from what).
- Avoid figurative, idiomatic, ambiguous language when presenting lessons.
- Give short, simple verbal instructions. Repeat and clarify by changing or redefining thc words and tcrms.
- Accompany verbal instructions with visual cues (underline keywords), clear diagrams to illustrate relevant information/concepts.
- Where possible, give practical demonstrations.
- Give information in small chunks. Daniel may have difficulty processing a lot of information at one go. Review often.
- Slow the pace/speed of the lesson.
- Alert Daniel to the important topic or concept being taught. For example, "I am going to tell you a story and then we will discuss WHERE it takes place".
- Talk slowly, with brief pauses after keywords. Put emphasis on key phrases or new ideas.
- Provide a brief written outline of points that may be covered in discussion. Stop part-way for summation of the discussion to that point. A written point summary could be provided at the end of the discussion.
- Provide extra assistance to Daniel to start a task. Outline the first step for him. Check that he has started.

George, Age 8 Years, Enrolled in Year 3

George was a victim of a hit-and-run car accident. He sustained a significant traumatic brain injury with left frontal lobe contusions and a midline shift. His teacher referred George to me because he was highly distractible in class and had significant difficulty concentrating on any set activity. George had a tendency to get out of his seat and wander the classroom whenever the work appeared to be too challenging for him. He was not like this before his accident.

An assessment by the school counsellor on the WISC-IV revealed that George was functioning within the average range of general intelligence with working memory deficits. There was no significant difference between verbal and nonverbal modalities.

Table 8.2 George's profile of strengths and weaknesses from the FES

Domains	Strengths	Weaknesses
Emotional/behavioural	Relates well to peers	
Metacognitive	No issues with planning skills	Difficulty following class rules
		Concentration problematic
		Highly distractible
		Working memory deficit

George's teacher completed the Functional Executive Scale (FES), and his profile was contained in Table 8.2.

I sat down with George and explained the results of his profile on the FES. I asked him whether he was aware that he was having problems focusing on the work. His teacher had told me that he would constantly get out of his seat and that he had problems sticking to his school work. Was this something that he would want to work on so that he had a chance to do well with his classwork? The added benefit would be that he would not get into so much trouble from his teacher. I told him that perhaps I could help him to achieve these goals as I had some influence with his teacher. George agreed to work with me in the classroom. I told him that it was not going to be easy and that he would have to work hard to break the habit but that if he was really serious, I believed we could do it together. I explained that I had helped other children who were having similar problems.

The first thing we needed to do was to develop a plan that George could follow to stay on task and not be so easily distracted in the classroom. I asked him to tell me what he did when he was at home, what he liked doing for fun. He said that he played on his XBox with friends. He told me about the games that he played. He described one game called Minecraft which he really enjoyed playing. It contained Lego characters where players can create their own world. I asked him how long he thought that he played Minecraft without losing concentration. He thought he stuck at it for about an hour before losing concentration. I subsequently confirmed this with his mother.

So, the evidence was that in one situation George could focus for an hour on a computer game and in another situation at school he had limited concentration. We needed to apply those concentration game skills to his school work. How could we do this? And was it just lack of motivation to his school work that was the issue at school?

I decided to work with George to develop a metacognitive strategy that would bring in some of the elements of his computer game. That was the skill we needed to draw on and apply to his school work. We talked about elements of Minecraft. What did he find so interesting that held his attention for so long? He liked the Lego characters, particularly the character Alex and the fact he was free to create his own structures. Okay, so Lego was a big motivator. We could use Lego characters in his plan.

The metacognitive strategy we both agreed on was the following:

LISTEN!
FOCUS.
WHERE ARE YOU UP TO?
ALEX CAN HELP YOU FINISH YOUR WORK.
YOU DID IT!

George's teacher was involved in the development of the plan and agreed that George could be rewarded if he increased the amount of time he was able to stay on task and stay in his seat. I worked with George in the classroom teaching him how to use the plan which I had printed out and placed on his desk. The printed plan included a picture of ALEX, his superhero, to remind George that with the help of Alex he was able to do this. I wandered around the classroom helping other children as well, and whenever his teacher noticed that George was being distracted or out of his seat, he would give a signal to George. The teacher would say "Class Listen!" and make eye contact with George. He would then approach George and tell him to look at his Plan, to focus on what he was doing and ask him where he was up to with his work. I would then step in and encourage George to follow the steps of the plan. I would get him to draw on his superhero Alex and tell him that Alex would be proud of the work he was doing by staying on task and finishing his work.

The teacher kept a record of the number of times George got out of his seat and the number of times he had to alert George to stay on task. This was charted at the end of each day, and George was given a reward if there was improvement. He got to choose the reward from a list the teacher had prepared.

The takeaway from this case study was that you need to delve into the background of younger children in particular and find something that they can draw on for strength or inspiration. What do they do for fun? Who are their heroes? Let's use these superheroes to encourage them to improve their functioning and be like their heroes—successful, powerful, doing the right thing and following the rules. You can draw on the imagination of these young children and incorporate their superheroes into their metacognitive plans.

Frank, Age 23

Frank sustained a significant traumatic brain injury following a motor vehicle accident. He sustained a fractured frontal bone, contusions to the right temporal lobe and a severe bleeding on the brain which needed to be evacuated. An assessment revealed dysexecutive function, poor memory and poor motivation. Frank had lost his job prior to his accident and was unmotivated to look for work. Frank lived on his own in a granny flat on his father's property in a small regional town. Frank no longer drove. He was on unemployment benefits and tended to spend most of his money on cigarettes and alcohol during the first week and had little money for basics to last the second week. He would constantly go to his father for financial assistance. Frank needed to get around the town by public transport although often had no money to pay for the local bus service.

My role was to work with Frank to assist him to manage his day-to-day affairs—budgeting, shopping, travelling and involving him in a work-related activity—not an easy task given his entrenched behaviour and poor motivation.

I first approached the issue of budgeting. Frank's welfare payments went directly into his bank account every 2 weeks. On pay day his normal course was to immediately go to the supermarket and buy cigarettes and alcohol using his card or cash. I sat down with Frank and worked out a reasonable budget with him. We itemised what his commitments were, how much he should spend on shopping and what he could afford vis-à-vis cigarettes and alcohol. He agreed to place a limit on these items. We worked together to draw up a plan that I placed into a mind map which he would keep in a prominent place as a reminder.

However, how could you encourage Frank to keep to this commitment? I approached the one and only supermarket in the town and, with Frank's approval, made an agreement with them. Frank had agreed to place a limit on his spending of cigarettes and alcohol. I drew up a contract which we both signed and was countersigned by the supermarket manager. The supermarket agreed that they would keep a record of his spending and advise him when he had reached that limit. The supermarket kept a copy of the signed contract to show Frank when he objected to their refusal to sell him anymore of the limited items. And there were a number of occasions during the early days when it came to that.

I did the shopping intervention program with Frank.

I would have liked Frank to quit smoking but I was going to choose my battles with him.

The next item was the transport issue. I approached the local bus company and made an agreement with them regarding Frank's transport. If Frank did not carry money for the ride, then they agreed to keep a record of the number of trips and cost and send a bill to his father at the end of each week. Frank's father was well-known and respected within the community. Frank agreed to repay his father. Frank used the bus service to go shopping and to go into town to meet his friends.

I then turned to involving Frank in some form of community service or volunteering as a precursor to finding paid employment. This task was much more difficult. There were limited opportunities in the town and further limited by the fact he did not drive. Frank had previous work experience in hospitality working in a kitchen. However, he had a poor work history before his accident. We decided that he may be interested in volunteering in an aged care facility in their kitchen. I helped Frank put together a resumé which we sent off to two aged care facilities in the area. Both were accessible by the local bus company.

One of the aged care facilities agreed to a work trial. I had indicated to them that I was willing to provide on-site support to assist Frank to settle into the position. They agreed after they met me. Frank had a 2-week paid work trial. It was not a good start when he failed to turn up on the first day. On the second day, I met Frank at his house and together we travelled on the bus to work. We went through the structure of the day and his duties as a kitchen hand in the aged care kitchen with the head cook. I listed, in order, Frank's duties and the rough time for each task. I wrote this out on a chart for him and it was included in the mind map which we drew together.

I worked with Frank every second day over the 2-week trial prompting him to follow the chart. Unfortunately, he was not offered the job. I suspected that he may have sabotaged the work trial.

I continued to work with Frank over a period of 6 months. He eventually did keep to his budget and cut down on his alcohol and cigarette intake. He went shopping regularly and caught the bus. I am uncertain whether he actually repaid his father for the bus fares. I was not successful in finding him employment or volunteering although given his premorbid poor work history I knew it would be a challenge. I later learned that he found a part-time job as a labourer in a mine where his father was a foreman (Fig. 8.1).

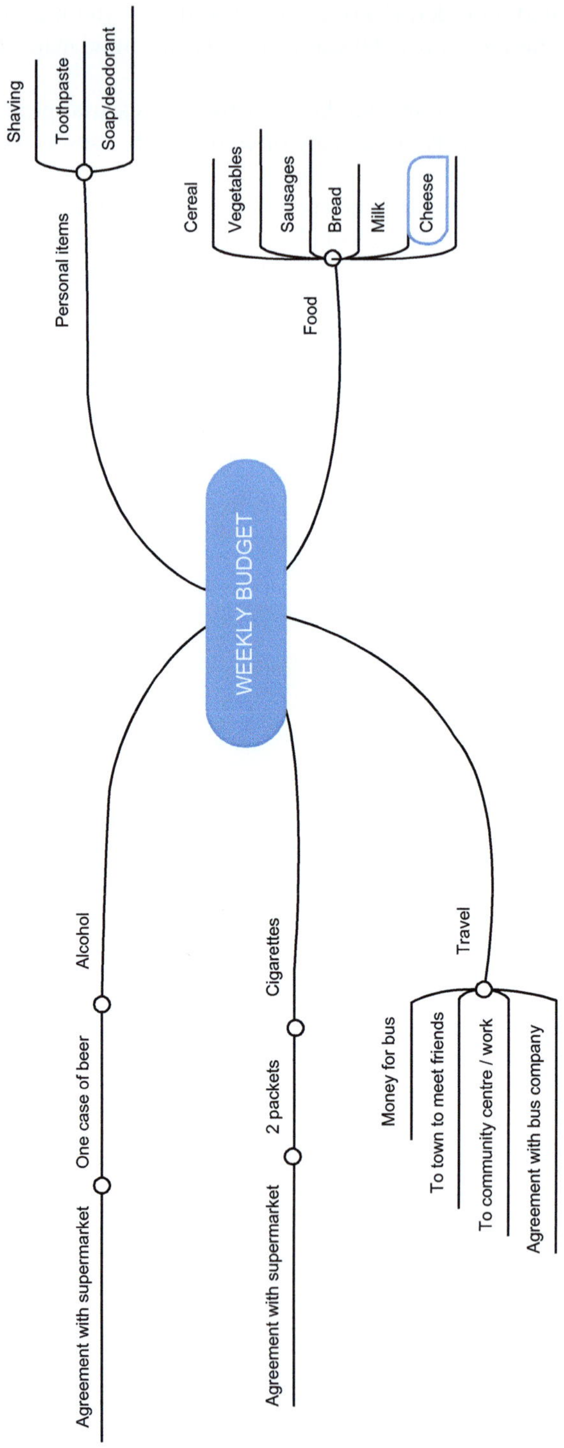

Fig. 8.1 Frank's mind map

Chapter 9
Memory

According to Fuster (1993), executive function is the interaction between working memory and planning processes, two mutually complementary cognitive functions. He opines that both functions are critical to bridging the gap between perception and action. It is part of his perception-action cycle and is consistent with the view that a primary competency of the dorsolateral prefrontal cortex is the integration of memory and inhibitory control.

There is evidence of a double dissociation between working memory and planning skills. Tasks that draw upon only one of these skills, such as the delayed non-match to sample task that makes use of only working memory, can be successfully solved by monkeys. According to Diamond (1990), evidence is also presented that tasks which utilise response inhibition skills, but not working memory skills, do not involve frontal lobe functioning.

To further illustrate this divide between working memory and planning/action, consider the case of clients with traumatic brain injury and executive dysfunction who can often tell you what they need to do although have difficulty bridging the gap between knowing and doing. In between knowing and doing is distractibility, inflexibility, lack of initiation and disinhibition. Often this is an issue primarily with working memory: keeping a goal in working memory so that you are moving toward achieving that goal without becoming distracted.

A picture is beginning to emerge which suggests that prefrontal cortex functioning involves more than just adaptive behaviour during novel and complex situations. Intact dorsolateral cortex is necessary in solving tasks which involve novelty and complexity. In solving these tasks, two independent and parallel dorsolateral neural systems are activated. These two systems appear to be integral to the successful resolution of executive or metacognitive functioning.

First, a goal must be established that is then retained in working memory during performance of the task. Then, planning must occur to establish the strategies and their sequence. Through the interaction of both working memory and planning, inappropriate responses are inhibited, new strategies are developed to meet the demands of the changing environment, and the individual remains on target to complete the goal.

J. Baron Levi, *The Hairy Bikie and Other Metacognitive Strategies*,
https://doi.org/10.1007/978-3-030-46618-3_9

So, what exactly is working memory? If I can use the analogy of a computer screen, working memory is what you have up on the screen in front of you at any one time. Perhaps you are writing and composing a piece of text directly onto your computer. Working memory, then, is what you are currently working on and seeing on the computer screen. When you scroll down from that screen to another page as it were, then it goes into short-term memory, and when you save what you have, it goes to long-term memory. Working memory, then, is the immediate conscious memory for what you are currently working on while you are manipulating information to achieve a particular goal or outcome. It is the capacity for temporarily holding information available for processing.

You rely on working memory when you are figuring out how to do a mathematical problem and at the same time recalling the formula or steps that you need to solve the particular problem. It involves the multiple processing of information—remembering what you are doing and at the same time remembering the rules or steps that you need to solve the particular problem or activity you are working on.

There are a number of tests of working memory: the Digit Span subtest from the Wechsler intelligence scales is one such example. It requires you to remember a sequence of digits of increasing length. In the second phase of the test, you are required to reverse the order of a second sequence of digits. So, in the reverse order phase, you not only have to hold in working memory the particular sequence, but you must also manipulate that information to reverse the order of sequences of increasing length.

The Working Memory subtest from the Wide Range Assessment of Memory and Learning—Second Edition, WRAML2 (Sheslow and Adams 2003), contains a list of words read out to the client who is instructed to respond with all of the animals first and then all of the nonanimals. In a more complex level of the same task, the client is given a different set of words and asked to respond with all of the animals in ascending order from smaller to larger and then all of the nonanimals in any order.

We know that clients with significant traumatic brain injury and subsequent executive dysfunction typically have problematic working memory skills.

How do you strengthen working memory and how do you compensate for a working memory deficit?

The approach I have always taken in relation to memory impairment is to identify the specific memory issue that the client is facing in their day-to-day life and to devise a program or strategy to ameliorate that particular problem in their lives. For me, it is never about memory training per se. However, I will address programs that have been developed to improve general memory functioning later in this chapter.

The first issue I addressed with my clients was to teach them to remember important information and appointments. Many would forget to turn up for appointments or forget to hand in an assignment. When I first began providing cognitive rehabilitation to my clients, I taught them to use a diary to remember important information such as appointments, when assignments were due and when to take medication. I would show my clients how to draw up columns for each of the important aspects of their lives and to write in when each important aspect was due. They were encouraged to carry their diaries around with them, so the diaries had to be small enough that they could do this. We bought a commercial diary that was 1 day to a page and then drew up the following columns:

Things to do today	Assignments/homework	Other

Down the side of each column would be the time of the day that each activity was to be carried out. Many of the students I worked with had issues with remembering to hand in assignments or homework on time. So the middle column was used more as an assignment and homework planner. I taught my students to plan out when they would spend time on working on their assignments to ensure they were completed on time. So, day 1 would be the day they were given the assignment. What preparation did they need? Write a list of what was required to complete the assignment. Move forward in the diary, and write down each day what will be needed to work on that assignment. Give plenty of time to have it completed. Move forward to the day it is due to hand in and write this in bold letters. Check each day to ensure you are working on schedule.

Each time I met with my client, I would ask them to go through their diary and report to me how it was working and whether we needed to make any changes.

For some clients I also included a section on *Thoughts*, a little like a thought diary. They were encouraged to write how they felt during that particular day, whether there was any particular event that impacted on them, any successes they had. I always encouraged them to focus on the positives that may have occurred during that day. This was particularly important for clients who lacked self-confidence or who suffered from anxiety.

Technology has significantly advanced since those early days in the 1990s when we used a paper diary. With the advent of smartphones, I would teach my clients to use the calendar with an auditory prompt as a reminder for appointments or important events or activities. A number of my clients still preferred to use a paper diary.

An Australian study by Lannin et al. (2014) involved subjects with traumatic brain injury in an 8-week training program in the use of an “off the shelf” personal digital assistant such as a Windows platform and HP Palm that had the features of an alarm, calendar, address book and camera and which excluded the telephone functionality. The authors were able to demonstrate that digital personal assistant use in an 8-week program with occupational therapy training decreased functional memory failures and caregiver report of frequency of forgetting in patients with acquired brain injury more than use of non-electronic aids. The experimental group continued to use the electronic devices even after the trial had concluded. One caveat was that the authors concluded that the use of the personal assistant was effective for discrete recall of particular tasks more so than an ability to compensate for executive dysfunction.

Many of my clients complained they could not remember where they left their keys or wallets and would spend wasted time searching the house for these items. This was a major problem for many of them. My wife and I had been given, as a present, some time ago, a serving dish in the shape of a fish. We decided that we would use the dish to place our keys and wallets and glasses in the dish which we kept in a prominent place in our house. It became known as our "fish dish". Whenever we arrived home, keys, etc. would go into the fish dish, and we always knew where to find them. Even when the dish broke and we purchased a new dish which was not in the shape of a fish, we continued to refer to it as our "fish dish".

So, I taught my clients to use a fish dish! Simple but effective and it worked for them. In no time there were numerous fish dishes being used in houses and apartments across Sydney and New South Wales!

The insurance companies who referred clients to us knew that we specialised in working with young people as our training and experience had been exclusively with children and adolescents. Every now and then, they asked us to see adults. One such case was a woman in her late 30s who had been the victim of a vicious bashing while working as a carer in a home for people with disability. We'll call her Fay. Fay not only sustained a significant traumatic brain injury but developed a fear of men. Fay lived with her young children and husband who was very supportive. He gave up his job to be her full-time carer. Fay would only have a female consultant working with her, a job for my wife who worked with me. Cheryl had a background in special education and had taught children and adolescents with a range of disability in special classes and special schools. She had also worked as a state-wide special education consultant for early intervention and at one time had been a principal of a school for children with severe and profound disability. She was eminently qualified to provide rehabilitation.

Fay had problematic memory which was of concern as she would constantly forget to turn off the stove after cooking for her preschool child.

The first task was to eliminate the danger of the stove. Cheryl collaborated with Fay and her husband, and together they came up with a plan. It was simple but effective. Cheryl designed a sign that was placed above the door of the kitchen in a very prominent position (Fig. 9.1).

Cheryl visited Fay during meal time and prompted her to look at the sign and to ensure that the stove had been turned off. Her husband was very much involved, and he also encouraged Fay to check the sign. It took six or seven visits and prompting for Fay to get into the habit of checking the sign and ensuring that the stove had indeed been turned off. We left the sign up for a period of 3 months before Fay was confident that she would remember to turn off the stove. During that time we phased out the various steps, and by the end of the 3 months, we just had the picture of the stove as a prompt for Fay to remember to turn it off. The picture continued to stay there as a constant reminder although by that time Fay had internalised the steps and was independent in ensuring that the stove had been turned off. We believe the intervention program was successful because of the support and encouragement Fay received from her husband.

We received a referral for another young woman who had a significant brain injury. She lived with her father who cared for her. Joan was the case I had earlier mentioned who had difficulty remembering the sequence of clothing to put on when dressing and often would put her bra on last over her clothes. Cheryl worked with Joan and took a series of photos of the sequence of items of clothing in order. She then placed these photos on a chart which was hung on Joan's bedroom wall. Cheryl

Fig. 9.1 Fay's memory prompt

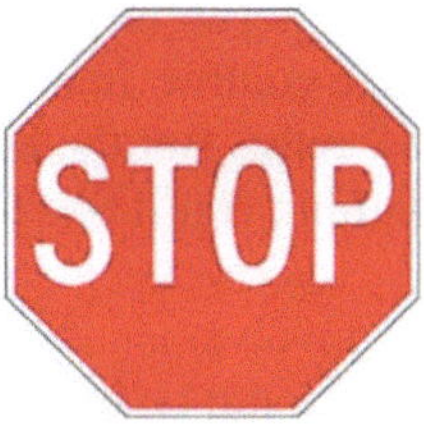

STOP!

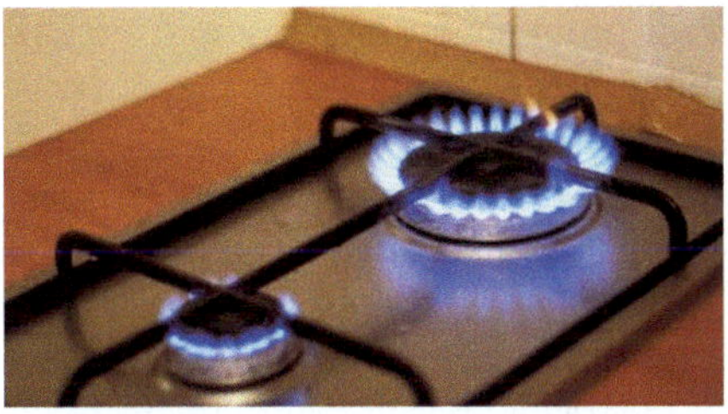

HAVE YOU TURNED OFF THE STOVE?

CHECK!

TURN OFF

TAKE THE POTS OFF THE STOVE

would then prompt Joan to follow the sequence. Eventually Joan was able to follow the sequence and dress herself appropriately.

We then collaborated with Joan and her father in setting a number of goals for Joan. Our main goal was to encourage Joan to get out into her community. We identified that shopping would be a realistic goal to begin with. Joan had a significant memory impairment. Joan's father would make up a list of shopping for the week. We decided that we would start with the goal of Joan going out to the supermarket and doing the shopping for her father. We would train Joan to do the shopping from the list. Cheryl accompanied Joan to the supermarket, a short distance from her house. This in itself was an issue because Joan would easily become lost and forget where she was. Cheryl drew a simple map for Joan to follow.

Once at the supermarket, they identified each of the items on the list and grouped them according to their location. So, all of the items in a particular shopping aisle were identified along with the aisle number and location.

Alongside each item was a box which Joan could tick when collected from the particular aisle. Cheryl printed this list out and made a number of copies.

Cheryl made up a diagram of the aisles and had this printed to assist Joan to navigate the supermarket to find her particular items. At first Cheryl accompanied Joan and prompted her to check her list. She would not find the items for Joan but encouraged her to look at the list and the location of the item. After a number of visits to the supermarket, Cheryl then began to shadow Joan, staying a few metres behind her and allowing Joan to take control. Joan was instructed that if she became stuck, she could call on Cheryl to assist. But the assistance was in the form of prompting and asking "Where do you think you'll find that item? Check the diagram. Show me where that is".

Cheryl phased down her involvement with the shopping program after 4 months once we were confident Joan could be independent in shopping.

Jack, 50 years old, had been referred to our employment service to assist him to find sustainable work. Jack had been an alcoholic over a long period of time and, as a consequence, had lost his family, his business and his home. The alcoholism left Jack with problematic memory and organisational issues. He also suffered from depression. There was no suggestion, however, that he had been diagnosed with Korsakoff's syndrome.

Jack had recently completed a Certificate III in Hospitality/Cooking at TAFE College and was interested in finding work as a cook. He enjoyed cooking. Cheryl worked with Jack and after gaining his trust began to promote him to local preschools who had a kitchen which provided meals for the children. This was considered an ideal slow-paced environment for Jack as he would not have been able to cope in a fast-paced stressful environment such as a cafe. There was also the issue of remembering orders, which Jack would have found challenging.

Cheryl eventually found a preschool willing to take Jack on. She and Jack visited the preschool and discussed the issues that Jack would experience on the job and gave assurances that Cheryl would work on-site with Jack and collaborate with the preschool director.

The first thing that Cheryl did was to collaborate with Jack and the director in drawing up charts and proformas covering:

- Details of the meals and snacks that needed to be prepared and delivered to each room at certain times
- Preparation times for each meal or snack
- A weekly menu planning proforma including budgetary information and a shopping list
- Individual dietary needs

Cheryl went on-site and helped Jack set up the program.

After a while the director called Cheryl and commented that Jack was sticking well to the routine and had become a grandfather figure to the children. She was happy to have him there although there was just one concern. The kitchen was getting messy and he was leaving his cleaning to the end of the day. Cheryl had a meeting on-site with Jack, and together they rejigged one of the charts to include time for cleaning up along the way.

The director reported that it was working very well and she was happy to have Jack at the preschool as good preschool cooks were hard to find.

Research on Memory Training

There has been much interest in training clients to improve their memory performance. The issue for a number of research studies was whether a particular successful working or prospective memory strategy taught in one context would transfer or generalise to another context.

In a recent article, Chan et al. (2019) noted that previous training studies had produced little evidence for transfer across contexts. The authors conducted a study involving 65 typically developing 6–9-year-olds in 3 training conditions and 1 control group: One group received rehearsal training, another group received semantic training, and a third group received training in both strategies. The rehearsal training involved recoding visual information into verbal information and then maintaining that verbal information in temporary storage through rehearsal. The semantic training group involved children thinking in terms of categories and deciding which object in a group did not belong with the others. Far-transfer or generalisation effects were assessed using a novel problem-solving task that was qualitatively different from the task on which children were trained.

The authors concluded that strategy-based training produced a far-transfer effect in a novel problem-solving task. There was no statistical difference in receiving combined training of both strategies compared to only one strategy. The authors concluded that future studies should be conducted to determine whether long-term gains can be produced by this type of working memory training.

In an earlier study, Turley and Whitfield (2003) involved undergraduate students in three types of working memory training: a rehearsal strategy, an imagery strategy and a semantic strategy. The authors concluded that those participants who had a low working memory ability as measured by pre-testing significantly increased their working memory span scores on the post-test when they were taught to use the rehearsal strategy. The effectiveness of imagery and semantic strategy training was less clear.

Bailey et al. (2014) trained older adults to use a working memory strategy when learning a list of words. The authors stated that age-related changes in brain integrity could result in slowing of information processing speed or in the ability to inhibit no longer relevant or task-irrelevant information from working memory. The mnemonic training involved both a visual and a verbal strategy—subjects were taught to use interactive imagery and sentence generation in a free recall of word lists. The results indicated that effective verbal encoding strategies benefitted working memory performance. However, the authors were not able to demonstrate transfer of the strategies to other working memory contexts.

Brain Training

I wanted to briefly raise the issue of computerised brain training which, according to van Heugten and colleagues (2016), is both topical and controversial. It wasn't that long ago our television screens were filled with advertisements for computerised programs that claimed to enhance brain functioning. According to Rabipour and Raz (2012), users in this field often relied on claims that were scientifically unsubstantiated.

van Heugten reported that for a therapeutic intervention to be considered clinically meaningful, it is necessary that the skills and behaviours developed in treatment transfer to nontreatment tasks and settings that are sustained following treatment termination.

Spencer-Smith and Klingberg (2015) conducted a meta-analysis of computerised training of working memory for inattention in everyday life using the Cogmed method. Of the 12 studies that met their inclusion criteria, the authors concluded that the major finding was that benefits of a working memory training program generalised to improvement in everyday functioning. However, the difference between the experimental and control groups was only 0.47 standard deviations, and long-term benefits 2–8 months after intervention were in the order of 0.33 standard deviations. The authors acknowledged that these were moderate improvements but nonetheless displayed improvement in working memory functioning.

According to Nouchi et al. (2013), a recent massive Internet-based research of adults aged 18–60 demonstrated that brain training games of certain types had no transfer effect on any other cognitive function. The authors conducted their own study using a commercial brain training video game and found that although a near transfer effect (immediate improvement effect) was demonstrated for executive functions and working memory, there were no far-transfer effects established (generalisation to cognitive domains unrelated to the trained cognitive processes).

It appears that a number of research studies treat working memory as if it were a separate entity. Baddeley (2002) asserts there is general agreement that memory cannot be regarded as a unitary faculty. In addition, the exercises used in the clinical studies cited were not necessarily real-world examples or problems. Subjects were typically involved in learning word lists or strings of numbers. Many of the studies were able to demonstrate improvement in working memory on one set of problems but unable to demonstrate generalisation or transfer to dissimilar problems. I also have not sighted any study that included a long-term follow-up of strategy use. The subjects in the studies I have quoted were neurotypicals. However, I acknowledge that the particular strategies in these studies may be useful when applied to real-work problems.

My view is that memory does not operate in a vacuum but is one component of a problem solving process. It needs to be incorporated in a broader problem solving or metacognitive strategy and applied to real-world problems. In that way, I believe there is a connectedness and relevance of working memory to the solution of a particular problem. How often in life, for example, do we need to learn a list of words or strings of numbers? In real life we need to remember where we left our keys, whether we locked the car, turned off the stove or the names of people we have just been introduced to.

My interest, for example, is in training a client with traumatic brain injury to negotiate a supermarket to find the targeted items they may have on their shopping list. There is a working memory component to this activity, but it is part of a larger problem solving task. The case study of Joan in this chapter is a case in point. The components of a shopping task for a client who has difficulty with shopping are as follows:

- They have to work out what items to place on the list. The list may come from the type of meals they wish to prepare for the week plus other general cleaning/laundry items. Write out the list, grouping items according to their food or grocery category.
- They need to find their way to the supermarket. Draw a map showing how to get there.
- They need to remember where each item is located on the supermarket shelf or to have a strategy for locating each item.

Each of these steps involves some memory component. I may use a visual and a verbal strategy to assist my client in this process. Together we may make up a small book for the client to follow. We may cluster items (semantic category) that group together, e.g. a separate category for dairy, meat, canned foods and laundry. We may then take pictures of each of these items or cut out pictures from the supermarket catalogue and paste them together on a diagram of each aisle in the shopping book. So, aisle 3 is the dairy section, and we have listed milk, cheese and butter and pasted pictures of these items on aisle 3. This becomes the visual strategy that the client can easily reference.

This begs the question. Having successfully taught my clients how to use this particular strategy when shopping, how likely are they to apply the same principle to another problem they may encounter? It may be at that point that I introduce the Hairy Bikie strategy and show them how the steps we followed in solving the shopping dilemma were the same process we would have used with the Hairy Bikie strategy. I may then go on to look at another issue they were facing and show them how to use the Hairy Bikie to solve that issue.

References

Baddeley, A. D. (2002). The psychology of memory. In A. D. Baddeley, M. D. Kopelman, & B. A. Wilson (Eds.), *The handbook of memory disorders* (2nd ed., pp. 3–15). West Sussex, UK: Wiley.

Bailey, H. R., et al. (2014). Does strategy training reduce age-related deficits in working memory? *Gerontology, 60*, 346–356.

Chan, S., et al. (2019). Far-transfer effects of strategy-based working memory training. *Frontiers in Psychology, 10*, 1285.

Diamond, A. (1990). The development and neural bases of memory functions as indexed by the AB and delayed response tasks in human infants and monkeys. In A. Diamond (Ed.), *The development and neural bases of higher cognitive functions* (pp. 267–317). New York: New York Academy of Sciences press.

Fuster, J. M. (1993). Frontal lobes. *Current Opinion in Neurobiology, 3*, 160–165.

Lannin, N., et al. (2014). A randomised controlled trial of the effectiveness of handheld computers for improving everyday memory functioning in patients with memory impairment after acquired brain injury. *Clinical Rehabilitation, 28*(5), 470–481.

Nouchi, R. et al. (2013). Brain training game boosts executive functions, working memory and processing speed in the young adults: A randomised controlled trial. *PLoS One*, San Francisco 8(2) February 2013.

Rabipour, S., & Raz, A. (2012). Training the brain: Fact and fad in cognitive and behavioural remediation. *Brain and Cognition, 79*, 159–179.

Sheslow, D., & Adams, W. (2003). *Wide range assessment of memory and learning* (2nd ed.). Florida: Psychological Assessment Resources.

Spencer-Smith, M., & Klingberg, T. (2015). Benefits of a working memory training program for inattention in daily life: A systematic review and meta-analysis. *PLOS One*. https://doi.org/10.1371/journal.pone.0119522.

Turley, K. J., & Whitfield, M. M. (2003). Strategy training and working memory task performance. *Journal of Memory and Language, 49*, 446–468.

van Heugten, C. M., et al. (2016). Brain training: Hype or hope? *Neuropsychological Rehabilitation, 5*(6), 639–644.

Chapter 10
Essay Writing

Students who have learning/executive function difficulties often find essay writing to be challenging. There is a sequence that needs to be followed in order to write a detailed and comprehensive essay or assignment. The students often do not expand on their ideas, do not necessarily follow a sequence to their writing and often miss the most important pieces of information that are provided.

In 1994 a journalist student who had been involved in a serious motor vehicle accident and sustained a significant traumatic brain injury was referred to our service. He returned to his university studies although he was experiencing difficulty with essay writing. His lecturers identified that when he was asked to write a five-page essay on a particular human interest story, he invariably handed in half a page. He had difficulty in expanding on his ideas and often was not aware of how to flesh out the main points of the topic.

So we worked together on developing an essay writing planner that he could use for any essay. What we came up with was a wheel that displayed the sequence of steps that he needed to work through to identify the topic and conduct the research so that he could identify at least five points that he would expand, and that each point would be a new paragraph or two. In 1994 the research involved going to the library and checking the CD-ROM machine! Figure 10.1 details the essay wheel we developed.

Over the years I refined the essay writer with a number of students who were experiencing similar issues with essay writing. What I eventually came up with was the WrAP.

WrAP

The Writing Assignment Planner (WrAP) is a planner that assists students in the planning, preparation and writing of an essay and/or assignment across a range of educational settings. It is intended to be used by students from primary/elementary

J. Baron Levi, *The Hairy Bikie and Other Metacognitive Strategies*,
https://doi.org/10.1007/978-3-030-46618-3_10

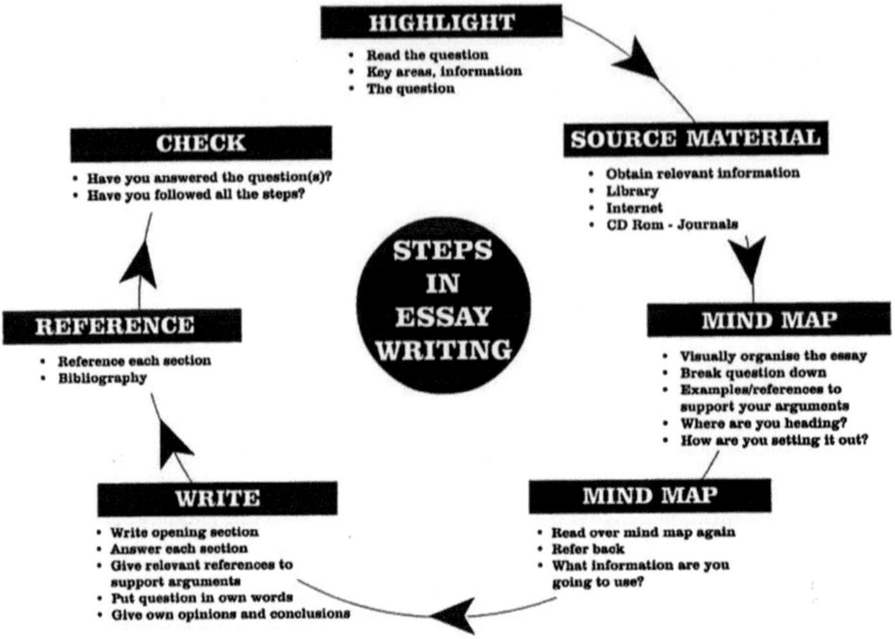

Fig. 10.1 Essay writing planner

level to tertiary settings as the underlying processes remain the same. Only the content and level of sophistication will change.

The WrAP is a writing planner which takes the student through a number of processes and routines in order to develop a visual plan of the essential elements of the particular writing project. The visual plan is then used by the student as a road map to write the essay/assignment.

Teachers of students with learning difficulty, whether as a result of a traumatic brain injury, autism or ADHD, would complain that students failed to expand on their ideas, failed to check that they had focused on the main points of the essay and failed to check the final draft of their essay.

The WrAP grew out of research and practice that the author developed to assist learners who were experiencing difficulty in understanding the questions, knowing what they had to do, knowing how or where to obtain the relevant information, knowing how to set out and sequence their response, knowing how to check or evaluate that they had answered the questions fully and that their response made sense within the context of the questions.

The WrAP model has been tested over a number of years directly with students at primary/elementary, secondary and tertiary levels and found to be an effective tool for those who required a structured approach to learning. It involves process-based learning, teaching students the underlying skills required to successfully complete a writing project or essay and assignment, on time, and using all of the available data. The steps in the WrAP are as follows see Fig. 10.2.

Fig. 10.2 WrAP Essay Planner

WrAP Content

Step 1: HIGHLIGHT

Read the question.
Highlight the important information and words.
What are you asked to do?
Define the terms/important words.
Make a list of the important aspects/parts of the question.
Do you understand what you have to do?
If not, ask for help.

Step 2: RESEARCH

Research the topic and the important terms/words.
Where can you find the information you need?
Are you sure this is the best approach?
How about using the Internet?
Summarise the important information.
Put it in your own words.

Step 3: PLAN

Write out a plan for how you will complete the essay/assignment.
Break the question down into smaller parts and plan each part.
Draw a visual plan/diagram of what you will include in your response.
Do you know how to present your response?
Who can you ask?

Step 4: WRITE

Write opening section.

Define the terms at the beginning of your answer so that the reader understands what you are talking about and you can show that you know what you are talking about. Answer each section in a separate paragraph.

Use the references from your research to support your arguments. Put your arguments in your own words.

Table 10.1 Example of evaluation proforma for the essay planner

	Not at all	For some of the time	For most of the time	All of the time
I was able to use the essay/assignment writer	1	2	3	4
I was able to complete the essay/assignment on time	1	2	3	4
I was realistic about the time it took to complete the assignment	1	2	3	4

Give your own opinions and don't be afraid to differ from the information you have read.

Don't be afraid to be critical or to give another opinion or point of view.

Summarise your arguments at the end of the essay/assignment.

Give a conclusion and maybe suggest "Where to from here?" for future action on this topic. Do a spell check.

Step 5: REFERENCE

Make sure you have included all of the references you used and in the right format.

Step 6: FINAL CHECK

Read over your work for a final check. Does it make sense? Have you answered the question? Did you include all of the information you were given? Did you include all of the references you gathered? Did you write it within the word limit and in the correct format? Ask someone to read your response.

Step 7: EVALUATION

Complete the evaluation sheet (Table 10.1).

WrAP Essay Example

Describe five endangered animals of the African Savanna and illustrate why they face extinction.

Step 1: Highlight

Highlight the directives. The directives are the words which tell you how to address the topic or question. What are you directed to do? **DESCRIBE and ILLUSTRATE.**

So, let's highlight the directives in the essay so that we keep them in mind when writing the essay. We'll highlight them.

Describe five endangered animals of the African Savanna and **illustrate** why they face extinction.

Now, we will highlight the keywords in a different colour. What are the important keywords in the essay? We will highlight these.

Describe **five endangered** animals of the **African Savanna** and illustrate why they face extinction.

Step 2: Research
We need to be sure we understand the keywords, so first we will check their meaning. We can Google each word.

Endangered: A species whose numbers are so small that the species is at risk of extinction, or being wiped out completely, like the dinosaurs.
African Savanna: A rolling grassland dotted with trees found in East Africa. It has plants such as Bermuda grass and elephant grass and found in countries such as Kenya, Angola and Zambia.
Extinction: A species faces extinction when the last surviving member dies.

Look back at the highlighted keywords: We next need to research five endangered animals.

We can check with Google or the Internet to find five endangered animals of the African Savanna. Here is what I found: Grévy's zebra, black rhino, cheetah, African wild dog and African elephant.

Write a separate paragraph on each animal.

Step 3: Plan
I am going to draw a visual plan of the information I have gathered and then use this to further expand on my ideas. Below is my mind map of the information I will use to write my essay. See Fig. 10.3.

Step 4: Write
We can now go ahead and write up the essay using all of the information we have gathered and outlined in the mind map in Fig. 10.3. Each endangered animal in the circles above represents separate paragraphs.

First, we need to define the topic, so we start with a definition of the keywords so that the reader knows we understand what we are talking about, and then we lead into the topic of describing the animals and then explaining why they face extinction. It is important that you write the essay in your own words! Do not just copy straight from the Internet!

At the end of the essay, write a brief summary of your main points. Maybe you have an idea of how the particular animals could be saved from extinction. Maybe there are animal groups who are working to save these animals, and you could describe the work that they are doing and perhaps any successes they may have had.

Step 5: Reference
We need to reference where we found the information. Was it from a particular book you found on Google or from Wikipedia or from some other source? Make sure you include a bibliography or list of references in the format your teacher or lecturer expects of you.

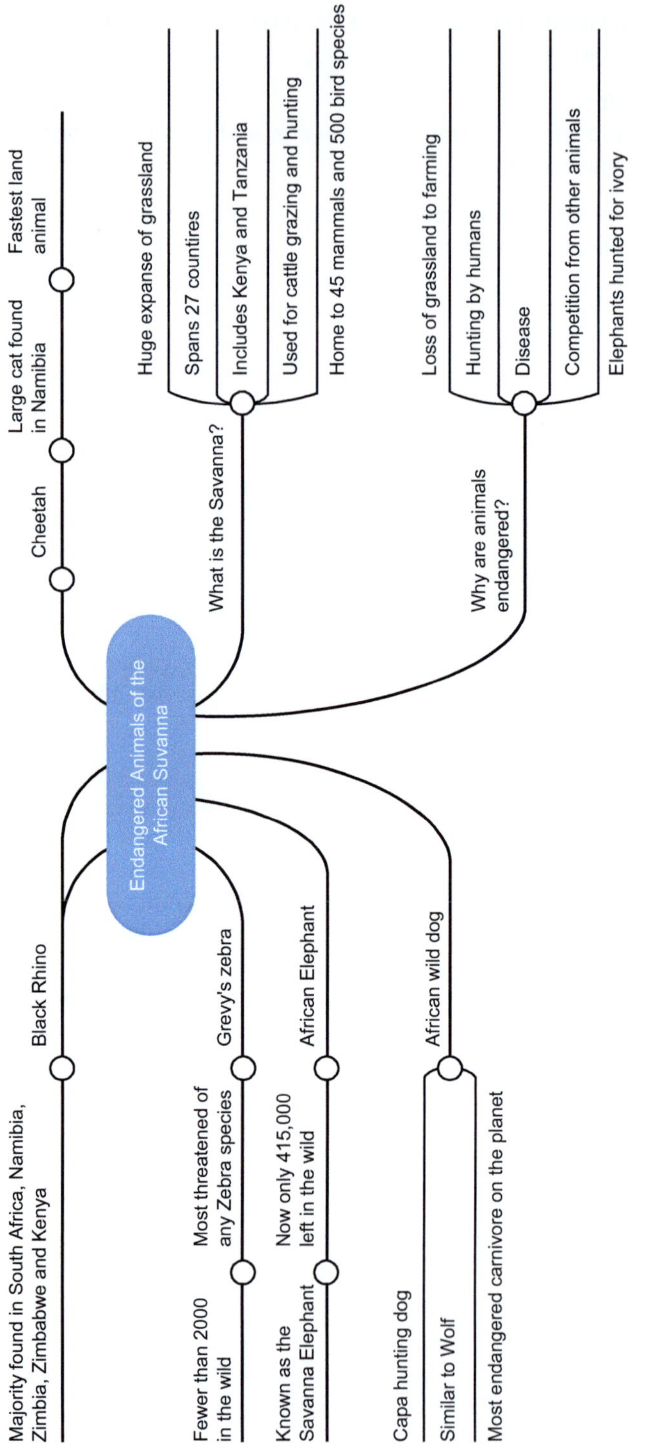

Fig. 10.3 Mind map of endangered animals

Step 6: Final Check

Read over your essay, check for spelling or grammar, and make sure you have answered the question. Well done!

Step 7: Evaluation

Complete the evaluation. How useful did you find the WrAP? Did it help you to expand on your ideas and put your essay into a sequence that made sense? Do you feel it saved you time that was not wasted?

Chapter 11
Anger Management

Anger management can be one of the most difficult areas in which to change behaviour. Challenging behaviours can be the hallmark of TBI, ADHD, CD, ASD or significant learning difficulty.

I implement a problem solver in conjunction with an approach to externalise the anger. In my experience the two approaches work well together.

"Externalising" is a concept that was first introduced to the field of family therapy by White and Denborough (1998). Initially developed from work with children, externalising has to some extent always been associated with good humour and playfulness (as well as thoughtful and careful practice).

There are many ways of understanding externalising, but perhaps White (1998) best summed it up in the phrase: "the person is not the problem; the problem is the problem". So, the issue or concern is phrased in a way which takes the blame away from the individual and places it on an external force.

When my wife was teaching preschoolers, she used to keep a "grump bucket" in her classroom. Before the children entered the classroom, she would, when appropriate, hang the grump bucket on the outside of the classroom and ask the children: does anyone have any grumps they need to get rid of today? We are not going to have any grumps enter our class today. Okay, place them in the grump bucket. This was done in a fun way, so she would go around and say: are you sure you are not hiding any grumps? Let me look behind your ears. There's one! In the bucket. They are pretty good at hiding, so you have to search carefully! Making it a playful activity actually helped the children to alter their mood and, consequently, their behaviour. The children would be asked to check other children for grumps so that it became a fun-filled playful activity.

Externalising involves asking questions in a way that invites people to personify problems. For example, when working with a young child who wants to stop getting into so much trouble, an externalising question might be: "How does that Mr Trouble manage to trick you?" or "When is Mr Trouble most likely to visit you?" Through these kinds of questions, some space is created between the person and the problem, and this enables the person to revise their relationship with the problem.

J. Baron Levi, *The Hairy Bikie and Other Metacognitive Strategies*,
https://doi.org/10.1007/978-3-030-46618-3_11

For example, it is very hard for a young child or young person to feel they have anything to offer in dealing with all the trouble that seems to surround them—but dealing with Mr Trouble is another matter!

So, when addressing the issue of anger management, I introduce the concept of Mr Trouble who appears to be taking control of the young person and leading them wherever Mr Trouble wants to go to get the person into more trouble. I would say: "It appears that Mr Trouble is in the driver's seat and leading you wherever he wants to go and deliberately getting you into trouble".

He is taking you on a merry ride and deliberately getting you into trouble. In order to defeat Mr Trouble, we must call on some powerful forces! You will need all of the help you can get. We need to enlist a support crew. Who do you have who can support you in defeating Mr Trouble? Your teacher? Your parents? Are you up for it? You will also need to build up your strength because Mr Trouble has got hold of you and he is not going to let go easily. He has been having so much fun watching you get into trouble. You will need to be strong to defeat him. What can you do to build up your strength? You can go running; make sure you have a healthy diet that builds up your strength. You will need all of this because Mr Trouble has been controlling you for a long time and to break free from him will require all of your strength and support.

The externalising narrative obviously is aimed at young children, but older students also relate to the general concept of externalising the behaviour although the language would be age-appropriate.

So, we have externalised the anger, and it is now a battle between the forces of good on the one side, which includes the young person, his family and his teacher, and the forces of evil which is represented by Mr Trouble (Fig.11.1).

Fig. 11.1 Mr Trouble

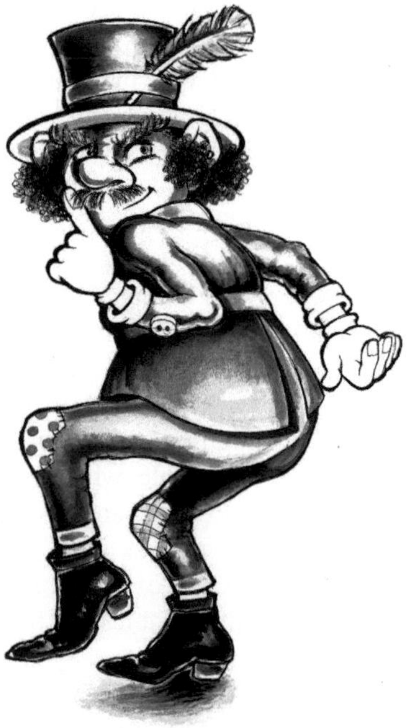

The support crew make a commitment to help the student defeat Mr Trouble, and they each make a pledge of how they will help and support.

One of the strategies I use in conjunction with Mr Trouble is a metacognitive approach that is developed in collaboration with the young person and the "support crew".

I teach strategies for remaining calm in anger-producing situations. What can you do to avoid conflict and Mr Trouble taking over? You can walk away. You can count to ten, do breathing exercises and calm yourself and tell yourself that you can remain in control and defeat Mr Trouble. You can also have a plan. At this point we work together to develop the metacognitive strategy.

A metacognitive strategy when you find yourself in a potential anger-producing situation would be:

STOP!
STAY CALM!
DON'T LET MR TROUBLE TAKE HOLD OF YOU!
I KNOW WHAT TO DO TO DEFEAT HIM—walk away, count to ten, breathe and say relax to yourself.
DO IT!
YOU DID WELL!

You can customise the externalising entity to fit any particular scenario. In Peter's example below, I used the concept of Mr Bossy for a child with ADHD who was being controlled by "Mr Bossy". In the case of poor behaviour, it was "Mr Trouble" who was leading the child into trouble. The young person you are working with may relate better to a "Mr Angry" (Fig. 11.2).

Fig. 11.2 Mr Bossy

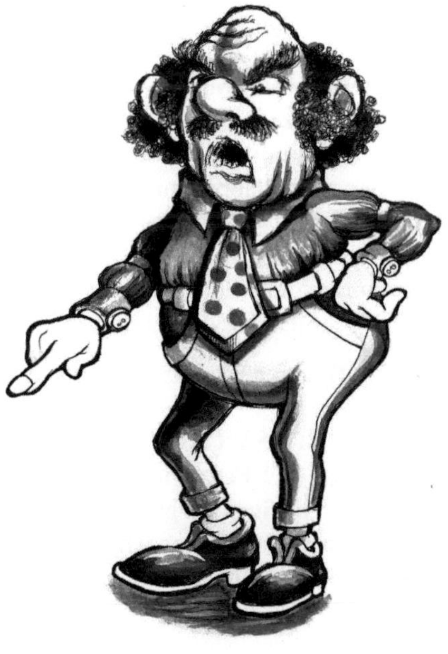

Peter's Rehabilitation Plan (from Chap. 5)

There were several aspects to Peter's rehabilitation plan. I had made recommendations for his teacher to consider, and then there was the direct intervention for Peter based on the results of the FES.

Notes for Peter's Teacher

Try to catch Peter out "being good". Take notice of him and praise him whenever you see him acting appropriately. Try to reinforce this type of behaviour rather than giving him attention whenever he is acting inappropriately. The general idea is that acting appropriately is incompatible with acting inappropriately.

If we identified that his acting out was in response to being unable to do the set work because of his learning difficulty, then he may need to be given work at his level or give him smaller chunks of work rather than overwhelming him with a lot of text. Once he has completed this section, then we can look at the next section.

I may try an externalising approach with Peter given that he is still in primary school and the approach would be age-appropriate. We identified from the FES that the emotional/behavioural aspect of executive function was of most concern in the classroom. He had difficulty following school and class rules and difficulty accepting criticism in addition to the poor behaviour. We know that with ADHD the issues are generally around lack of control of behaviour as well as impulsivity. So, there is an external somebody controlling his behaviour, taking control of him and pulling the strings. Who could that be? Let's call this person Mr Bossy because he is bossing you around and taking control of you.

We know you want to take back control of your behaviour from Mr Bossy, so we need to work out a way that he doesn't always control you and boss you around doing things that you don't want to do.

And so, like the concept of Mr Trouble, we build up a scenario of this external Mr Bossy taking the blame for Peter's behaviour.

I then, in collaboration with Peter and his teacher, develop a metacognitive plan for him to follow to defeat Mr Bossy and take back control of his behaviour. I ask Peter what he could do to take back control of his behaviour from Mr Bossy. We brainstorm some ideas and then write them down.

The problem solving plan was as follows:

STOP! Teacher signals to Peter when it is obvious that Mr Bossy has taken control.

LET MR BOSSY GO. Peter acknowledges that Mr Bossy has taken over.

I CAN DO IT! Peter practises strategies to defeat Mr Bossy. Peter engages in deep breathing and guided self-talk: "I can beat Mr Bossy. I can kick him right out of my life! I know what to do to beat him and stop him bossing me around. He doesn't want me to calm down but I will show him that I can do this!"

KEEP MR BOSSY AWAY. Peter goes back to doing his work and calms down. I DID IT!

Stress Inoculation Training

Another approach which I have used numerous times with older students and adults is Stress Inoculation Training developed by Donald Meichenbaum and Novaco and which I adapted to deal with anger management.

Stress Inoculation Training is a *cognitive-behavioural* approach providing people with added *psychological resilience* **a**gainst the effects of anger. The general principles of the anger control approach were developed by Novaco (1975).

The program usually comprises three phases:

- *The Conceptualisation Phase*—learning to conceptualise and reconceptualise anger. So we discuss "what is anger and where does it come from?" We are not born with anger—it is learned and therefore can be unlearned. What are the signs of anger? Can you feel anger? What does it feel like—can you recognise it? Can you rate it on a 10-point scale?
- *Skills Acquisition and Rehearsal Phase*—including problem solving, cognitive restructuring and guided self-dialogue. It is important to understand that anger cannot be effectively managed by adopting a "cookbook approach" but that triggers to anger need to be appraised and a range of coping options are available to the student who can decide how best to employ them.
- Once the young person recognises under what situations they become angry, I then teach different strategies for managing anger. Replace negative thoughts with positive ones. It is what you tell yourself that drives your behaviour.
- I gently challenge some of the irrational beliefs that my clients may harbour using Reality Therapy principles.
- So what if you make a mistake, will the world suddenly end? Mistakes are a learning experience. So what if he makes you mad—it is not your problem! Everything doesn't always have to go your way. Don't sweat the small stuff and it is all small stuff (Carlson 1997).
- Walk away from a situation that you know will get you angry. Stop and calm yourself—say **RELAX** quietly to yourself and do some deep breathing, feeling yourself relax.
- *Application and Follow-Through Phase*—Students are encouraged to write "coping contracts", monitor their behaviour and undertake homework in order to ensure responsibility for their own wellbeing. I develop a monitoring chart for students to track their behaviour and rate each one. Usually we focus on one or two behaviours that are of concern. The students show the chart to their teacher or parent at the end of each day.

An example of a monitoring chart may look like that in Table 11.1.

Table 11.1 Example of a behaviour monitoring proforma

Behaviour	Never	Sometimes	Often	Always
Losing my temper in class				
Talking back to teacher				

I then develop a Problem Solving Plan in collaboration with the student so that they use their own words to redirect their anger.

A typical metacognitive strategy may look like the following:

- STOP! I can feel myself getting angry and losing it!
- I DON'T HAVE TO GET ANGRY. So what if I make a mistake. I am still a good person. Does it really matter if he said that?
- I AM IN CONTROL. I know what to do to stay calm and in control. I can walk away from this because if I stay I will lose it. I know what signs to look for that I am about to lose my temper, and I know how to stop that.
- I CAN BE CALM. I can place myself in a calm place. I know how to do that.
- RELAX. Say "relax" to yourself. Feel yourself cooling down and your body losing its tension.

References

Carlson, R. (1997). *Don't sweat the small stuff. And it's all small stuff.* New York: Simon and Schuster.

Novaco, R. W. (1975). *Anger control: The development of an experimental treatment*. Lexington, KY: Lexington.

White, C., & Denborough, D. (1998). Companions on a journey: An exploration of an alternative community mental health project. In *Introducing narrative therapy: A collection of practice-based writings*. Adelaide, South Australia: Dulwich Centre Publications.

Chapter 12
Employment

The Supported Employment Model of Work Placement

The supported employment model of return to work began in earnest in the 1990s with Wehman et al. (1988) working with clients with severe disabilities. Although there has been a growing body of evidence to support the effectiveness of this approach not only in terms of job placement but job retention in the long term, evidence-based practices utilising this model of return to work have continued to lag. There have been variations of the supported employment model including Place-Train and Individual Placement and Support (IPS) both of which have specific variants. According to Corrigan and McCracken (2005), the Place-train model promotes rapid placement of people with acquired brain injuries (ABI) into a real job, followed by in situ support and training that assists the person to successfully remain in the job.

Burns et al. (2007) maintain that the research literature does not support the notion of work readiness as a prerequisite to a successful work outcome. What we do know from the literature is that traditional neuropsychological assessments, particularly clinical measures of executive function, are generally poor predictors of vocational readiness and success in employment. In one study Possl (2001) found that the success of clients despite a poor prognosis illustrated unsolved problems in relation to the ecological validity of neuropsychological measures of executive function. The researchers found 30% of the clients who tested with executive dysfunction were immediately and successfully placed in jobs that required skills mediated by intact executive functions in problem solving and organisational skills. In addition, research by Gallaher and colleagues (1998) has found that measures of injury severity as well as age were poor predictors of vocational outcome in a group of clients with ABI.

Standardised neuropsychological tests were never designed to assess a client's capacity to return to work or to function in the real world of work. Tests that are currently employed need to be adapted to provide more functionally relevant information. Baron Levi and Hartley (1992) present a view that neurobehavioural measures have more efficacy than standard neuropsychological measures.

J. Baron Levi, *The Hairy Bikie and Other Metacognitive Strategies*,
https://doi.org/10.1007/978-3-030-46618-3_12

The evidence suggests there should be less emphasis on injury severity and demographic characteristics and more on determining what type of service makes a good vocational outcome. Recent studies of clients with moderate to severe ABI by Cattelani et al. (2002) has shifted the focus from investigating the variables that may predict successful employment outcomes to investigating the type of vocational programs that will ultimately lead to successful and enduring job placements and improved quality of life.

Assessment in a place-train model is not for the purpose of screening clients or determining work readiness but to identify the type of support they would require on the job. It is for this reason that assessments need to be more functionally rather than clinically based. They need to measure a client's behaviour in a real-world setting and be based on observational data by the client and a person familiar with the client. The functional assessment tools then form the basis for baseline and ongoing continuous and comprehensive assessment while the client is in the workplace. Examples of such behavioural assessments have been used in research projects by Simpson and Schmitter-Edgecombe (2002).

The approach that I took with vocational rehabilitation involved the following features. An emphasis on ongoing assessment of workplace functional behaviours using a checklist specifically developed to measure executive function behaviours as they relate to the workplace. The Workplace Behaviour Assessment is completed by the client and the employer at regular intervals during the employment phase. This information is then used to provide feedback to the client so that necessary adjustments can be made and on-site intervention can be specifically tailored to the client's needs.

Education of the client following initial assessment of their strengths and weaknesses. This process was aimed at promoting self-awareness of the client's strengths and limitations and prepared them for the need to provide on-site job coaching that addressed the deficits in a real-world situation.

Job coaching involved metacognitive strategies which were specifically developed for each client. Job coaches were psychologists with a deep understanding of ABI and who had undergone a training program. Clients with executive dysfunction and memory impairment were trained to use a Problem Solving Plan as a compensatory strategy to increase their level of independence in the workplace. Problem Solving Plan represented a metacognitive strategy of a routine of knowing what it was that you had to do, working out a strategy for doing it, staying focused until you have completed the activity and then checking that it worked. Clients were coached on the job, to use the Problem Solving Plans as a form of frontal lobe prosthesis. Experience had shown that in time clients internalised the strategies and became independent in dealing with complex instructions and routines that may arise in the course of their work.

Assessment

The following assessment tool was used once the client was referred to the service:

Workplace Behaviour Assessment was completed by the client and a family member/case manager familiar with the client.

Workplace Behaviour Assessment©Jeffrey Baron Levi (2009)

Metacognitive	**0. Never occurs** **1. Sometimes occurs** **2. Often occurs** **3. Always occurs**	**Comment**
1. Aware of own limitations/disability	0… 1… 2… 3…	....
2. Can follow rules of a task	0… 1… 2… 3…	....
3. Is easily distracted by events around him/her	0… 1… 2… 3…	....
4. Can work independently	0… 1… 2… 3…	....
5. Is organised in his/her approach to work tasks	0… 1… 2… 3…	....
6. Can concentrate and attend to a task for an appropriate period	0… 1… 2… 3…	....
7. Able to start on a set activity without assistance	0… 1… 2… 3…	....
8. Completes tasks within a reasonable time frame	0… 1… 2… 3…	....
9. Becomes easily distracted during a task	0… 1… 2… 3…	....
10. Copes with changes in routine	0… 1… 2… 3…	....
11. Able to follow all steps of a particular activity	0… 1… 2… 3…	....
12. Anticipates consequences/thinks ahead	0… 1… 2… 3…	....
13. Can learn new information easily	0… 1… 2… 3…	....
14. Shows awareness when doesn't understand an activity	0… 1… 2… 3…	....
15. Able to learn from mistakes	0… 1… 2… 3…	....
16. Keeps appointments on time	0… 1… 2… 3…	....
17. Can make inferences and draw conclusions	0… 1… 2… 3…	....
18. Has good problem solving skills	0… 1… 2… 3…	....
19. Monitors behaviour and can self-correct	0… 1… 2… 3…	....
20. Gets stuck on certain activities	0… 1… 2… 3…	....
21. Seeks help if gets stuck on an activity/task	0… 1… 2… 3…	....
22. Seeks help if doesn't understand the task	0… 1… 2… 3…	....

23. Is realistic in the duties he is capable of performing	0…	1…	2…	3…	....
24. Can recall information taught the day before	0…	1…	2…	3…	....
25. Able to attend to/concentrate on an activity	0…	1…	2…	3…	....
26. Can remember and follow a sequence of tasks	0…	1…	2…	3…	....
27. Can remember information told to him/her	0…	1…	2…	3…	....
28. Has a strategy for remembering important information	0…	1…	2…	3…	....
29. Has better recall when prompted or cued	0…	1…	2…	3…	....
30. Remembers to bring materials to a meeting/activity	0…	1…	2…	3…	....
31. Always asks for instructions to be repeated	0…	1…	2…	3…	....
Behavioural/emotional					
32. Relates well to co-workers/peers	0…	1…	2…	3…	....
33. Can control his behaviour	0…	1…	2…	3…	....
34. Maintains a positive attitude toward work	0…	1…	2…	3…	....
35. Fatigues easily	0…	1…	2…	3…	....
36. Appears confident in social/work situations	0…	1…	2…	3…	....
37. Is motivated to engage in activities	0…	1…	2…	3…	....
38. Aware of own limitations	0…	1…	2…	3…	....
39. Aware of others' feelings/viewpoint	0…	1…	2…	3…	....
40. Shows appropriate emotional response toward co-workers/peers	0…	1…	2…	3…	....
41. Can graciously accept criticism	0…	1…	2…	3…	....
42. Able to make and maintain appropriate eye contact	0…	1…	2…	3…	....
43. Able to position himself at an appropriate distance in conversation	0…	1…	2…	3…	....
44. Able to control the volume and amount of own talk	0…	1…	2…	3…	....
45. Able to control his anger in the workplace	0…	1…	2…	3…	....

The Place-Train-Remain Model of Supported Employment (Baron Levi 2009)

The Place-Train-Remain model of placement of jobseekers with disabilities promotes rapid placement of people with disabilities into a real job, shared decision-making followed by in situ support and training that assists the person to successfully remain in the job. I added the "remain" component to ensure that jobseekers remained in sustainable employment by coaching them to become independent in the workplace through training on using a metacognitive strategy.

Place-Train-Remain promotes work as an immediate goal for a jobseeker who had been out of work for an extended period. A job search program is normally implemented within one month of the referral and is based on jobseeker preference and results of job interest and skill level.

The evidence suggests that the Place-Train-Remain model is significantly superior in outcomes compared to preparation or readiness Train-Place models which are based on moving jobseekers through a continuum from segregated to inclusive settings.

There is evidence that vocational outcomes in terms of job retention using a supported employment model such as the Place-Train-Remain approach can be improved with the addition of a social skills or cognitive training program specifically designed and developed for job tenure. We know that job retention involves skills in getting along with others for an extended period of time and that there is a relationship between social and vocational functioning. Most of the traditional vocational rehabilitation programs view accommodations to the workplace in terms of technical changes to the job tasks and routines and ignore the fact that accommodation to the workplace is really a social process. A training module designed to improve the social skills necessary for getting and keeping a job would include how work changes participants' lives, using problem solving to manage symptoms and medications at the workplace, how to deal with customers, how to deal with criticism from a supervisor and how to deal with stigmatising attitudes from co-workers. The social skills programs can be delivered off-site or on-site at the workplace using trained job coaches.

We know that many jobseekers with disabilities often present with problem solving difficulties and memory impairment, and these deficits are often associated with poor vocational outcomes. There is evidence that training jobseekers, on-site, to use a Problem Solving Plan or metacognitive strategy, as a compensatory strategy, can lead to an increase in their level of independence in the workplace. Jobseekers are coached on the job to use the Problem Solving Plans as a form of compensatory strategy either through an identified mentor or through post-placement support staff. Experience has shown that in time jobseekers internalise the strategies and become independent in dealing with complex instructions and routines that may arise in the course of their work. Problem Solving Plans have been successfully used with jobseekers with disabilities for many years. The metacognitive strategy forms the third phase of the Place-Train-Remain model.

Case Studies That Illustrate the Place-Train-Remain Approach to Return to Work

David

David was a 36-year-old who lived in Sydney and was struck by a motor car in 2009 while crossing the road and as a result sustained a significant injury. He had a compound skull fracture and physical injuries which restricted his return to work. David presented as agitated and distressed with significant stress symptoms on a formal mood questionnaire. There had been issues with anger management post-accident. The disability employment provider liaised with David' s psychiatrist on an ongoing basis to ensure that David's program was not contra-indicated by the medical evidence and to ensure that medical treatment and the employment program were "on the same page".

David was referred to the employment provider 2 years after his accident. Following initial assessment of David's memory functioning, workplace skills and behaviour using the functional assessment tools, a return to work plan which included pre-vocational and vocational activities, was developed. David was involved in an Anger and Challenging Behaviour (ACB) workshop, based on the principle of stress inoculation, to address his anger management issues. This was a 10-hour individual workshop providing David with an *educational* phase on causes and symptoms of anger, an *intervention* phase providing David with the behavioural skills to deal with his anger in a safe way and an *evaluation* phase to evaluate and adjust his responses to anger. David reported a diminution of his anger after the completion of the 10-hour workshop. David was encouraged to focus on his abilities and to look for opportunities to promote his abilities. David was encouraged to keep a thought. Diary and his personal entries were used as the basis for discussion and the opportunity to teach David to dispute his negative perceptions.

David had been working as a handyman prior to his accident, and an approach to his previous employer secured his old position although with reduced hours. David's case manager visited the work site and provided training and information to David's employer on the changes in David's behaviour due to his disability and to a range of strategies to manage David if he became agitated or frustrated at work. David's case manager worked with David and his employer using a Problem Solving Plan to compensate for his reduced working memory and problem solving capabilities. David was taught to use a diary and to write down important information. His employer agreed to provide David with simple written instructions and diagrams which David attached to his diary.

Because David was given set work to do each day that involved a regular routine of activities, the initial establishment of the program for him involved David being photographed actually doing each step of the routine. These photos were then placed on a board and in his iPhone, in sequence, as a ready reference for David to follow.

In addition, a simple Problem Solving Plan was developed in collaboration with David to assist him to follow the sequence of activities as illustrated in the photos to solve a particular work-related problem. The Problem Solving Plan was as follows:

- WHAT DO I HAVE TO DO?
- LOOK AT THE PHOTOS
- I KNOW WHAT TO DO
- DO IT!
- CHECK THAT IT IS CORRECT.

This plan was written on a chart for David to refer to. If his employer or work colleague noted that David was having difficulty with a particular task or appeared to be stuck, he would ask David where he was up to in his plan. David was then prompted to look at the photos and to continue to work through the steps to achieve an outcome. In time David internalised the plan and it became part of his thought process when solving problems. David remained in employment, and after 6 months his hours were extended to a full-time position. The Case Manager worked with David on-site for 4 months. During the time that David was working part-time, he came into the employment provider's office for continued support and discussions of his work experience so that any issues could be immediately dealt with by the Case Manager. David continued to remain employed in the same position.

References

Baron Levi, J. (2009). *Place train remain. A supported employment model of employment for clients with acquired brain injuries.* Paper presented at Annual Conference of Disability Employment Australia, Perth, Australia.

Baron Levi, J., & Hartley, P. (1992). A developmental and functional approach toward students with brain injuries. *The Australian Educational & Developmental Psychologist, 9*, 28–36.

Burns, T., et al. (2007). The effectiveness of supported employment for people with severe mental illness: A randomised control trial. *Lancet, 370*, 1146–1152.

Cattelani, R., et al. (2002). Competitive re-employment after severe traumatic brain injury: Clinical, cognitive and behavioural predictive variables. *Brain Injury, 16*, 51–64.

Corrigan, P., & McCracken, S. G. (2005). Place first, then train: An alternative to the medical model of psychiatric rehabilitation. *Social Work, 50*.

Gollaher, K., et al. (1998). Prediction of employment outcome one to three years following traumatic brain injury. *Brain Injury, 12*, 255–263.

Possl, J., et al. (2001). Stability of employment after a brain injury. *Brain Injury, 15*, 15–27.

Simpson, A., & Schmitter-Edgecombe, M. (2002). Prediction of employment status following traumatic brain injury using a behavioural measure of frontal lobe functioning. *Brain Injury, 16*, 1075–1091.

Wehman, P., Kreutzer, J., Wood, W., & Morton, M. V. (1988). Supported work model for persons with traumatic brain injuries: Toward job placement and retention. *Rehabilitation Counselling Bulletin, 31*, 298–312.

Chapter 13
The Research Project

The following is an abridged version of the article I wrote detailing the research project I designed and implemented in 1995 and 1996. I was awarded, in 1995, a 2-year research project funded by the then NSW Motor Accidents Authority to test out the efficacy of the Hairy Bikie problem solving plan. The project was titled *The HBMPC Problem-Solver: Training adolescents with traumatic brain injury to use a metacognitive approach to problem solving.*

The research involved 42 secondary students aged 13 to 15 years, who had moderate to severe traumatic brain injury as a result of a motor vehicle accident. All subjects had a Glasgow Coma Scale score less than 12 on admission to hospital. The students were randomly selected from a list of those who were admitted to the Children's Hospital at Westmead and the Sydney Children's Hospital at Randwick, who were at least 12 months post-injury and enrolled in mainstream secondary classes in Sydney. During the course of the research, five students dropped out of the study due to illness or transfer out of the area, so the next available subjects were included in the project. The 42 subjects completed the research.

The students were then randomly assigned to one of three groups: the cognitive training group (CTG), the placebo group (PG) and the control group (CG). The CTG and the PG were each involved in a 20-week individual intervention program that was delivered at the student's school. Fourteen students were placed into each of the three groups. Students in the CTG were taught to use the Hairy Bikie problem solving plan applied to their school work. The CTG self-monitored their use of the Hairy Bikie strategy in class.

The PG were involved in an individual 20-week intervention program that focused on reading comprehension exercises. The CG received no intervention.

All testing was administered by a research assistant who was blind to which group students belonged. Students were pre and post-tested on a range of cognitive and behavioural measures: the Child Behaviour Checklist, the Austin Maze, the Wisconsin Card Sorting Test, The Seals Test of executive function, self-monitoring charts as well as teacher observations of the students performing in the classroom.

J. Baron Levi, *The Hairy Bikie and Other Metacognitive Strategies*,
https://doi.org/10.1007/978-3-030-46618-3_13

Procedure

Cognitive Training Group

The CTG were given 20 individual weekly sessions of 45 minutes duration at their school. Students were withdrawn from class to participate in the program. The author delivered all the intervention. Teachers were not informed to which group students were assigned. Students were taught to use the Hairy Bikie (HBMPC) problem solving plan which was printed on labels for them to place at the back of all of their writing books. The protocols for each of the steps were also printed for the students to include in their work books.

The training sessions involved "informed training" where the students were explicitly told of the rationale and significance of the strategies and given responsibility for practising the skills in the classroom as per the method employed by Cicerone and Wood (1987). At the end of each session, students were led through a recap of strategies and processes used and given homework for the following session. During each session the HBMPC problem solver was applied to two types of problems: brain teasers and the student's own school work across the curriculum. The student's own work generally involved working on their homework in Mathematics, English and Science.

The author prompted the students to follow each step in the problem solving plan. Students were explicitly given information on using mapping to visualise the problem—a map could be a mind map, a timeline or a specific drawing. The author guided the students to use a faded cueing technique where they vocalised each step and talked through the steps they would take using HBMPC to solve the problem.

The students were also taught to monitor their use of the strategies at the end of each school day. They were given printed pro formas which they completed and brought to the next session to discuss their use of the strategies in the classroom.

Placebo Group (PG)

The PG received the same number of individual sessions for the same duration of time as the CTG—withdrawn for 45-minute individual sessions over a 20-week period. The PG was designed to control for the individual attention that students received during the intervention period.

The placebo intervention consisted of individual reading comprehension exercises which each student worked through with the trainer. It was contended that reading comprehension was a non-executive type activity where the students were not taught specific skills but simply given exercises to complete based on reading texts. Students were instructed to read a short story from a magazine or newspaper. A series of comprehension exercises were given to the student to complete. The stories were selected on the basis of their interest to a teenager and included sports and entertainment.

Control Group (CG)

The CG subjects received no intervention.

Pre-testing

The Seals Test – Baron Levi (1994)

This is an adaptation of the Tower of Hanoi. The test involved pictures of three seals each resting on a podium with coloured balls of varying sizes balancing on their noses. The subjects were to remember simple rules for moving the balls as well as the position of each ball. The rules for moving the balls were as follows: a larger ball cannot be placed on top of a smaller ball, you can only move one ball at a time and only move a ball from the top of the stack of balls. Subjects were required to plan further moves to solve problems within the minimum number of moves at three levels of difficulty: a two-ball problem (3 moves), a three-ball problem (7 moves) and a four-ball problem (15 moves). Subjects not only had to remember the rules for moving the balls but also keep in working memory the position of each ball as they "move" it. Each problem type involved six trials to completion, and subjects have to solve two successive trials for completion of that difficulty level. Whenever a subject violated a rule or made an incorrect move, the trial was terminated, and the balls moved one step closer to the target for the subject to begin at that particular point. The end target was always displayed at the top of each page.

The author had developed Australian norms for children from 7 to 16 years of age.

Wisconsin Card Sorting Test (WCST) – Nelson (1976)

This was a computerised adaptation of the WCST with the Nelson (1976) adaptation. The computer automatically scored the number of correct sets, time taken to complete the test, number of perseverative errors and total errors.

Austin Maze – Walsh (1985)

This is a computerised version of the Austin Maze. The dependent variables generated from the Austin Maze were total errors, number of trials to successful completion and time taken to complete.

Wechsler Individual Achievement Test (Screener)—WIAT – Wechsler (1992)

This is an individually administered test for assessing the achievement of children 5–19 years of age. The battery of tests contains basic reading, mathematics reasoning and spelling.

Test of Memory and Learning (TOMAL) – Reynolds and Bigler (1994)

The TOMAL is a comprehensive memory battery designed for children from 5 to 19 years. It is composed of a core battery of ten subtests (five verbal and five nonverbal) formally divided into a verbal memory scale and a nonverbal memory scale. A delayed recall procedure is also derived based on recall of stimuli for the first four subtests of the core battery and yields a delayed recall index.

Executive Functioning – Baron Levi (1994)

Class teachers completed the functional executive scale (FES). See Chap. 6 on assessment for a detailed explanation of the FES.

Results

The data for the 17 dependent variables was analysed using a Psy 32 for Windows 2.0 statistical package developed by Bird (1998). An issue in the analysis was the determination of a critical value for F. Given that there were 17 dependent variables, the possibility of type 1 errors loomed large. A decision was made to apply a rigorous method of controlling for type 1 error rate by applying a Bonferroni adjustment rate.

The Seals Test

From Table 13.1 it can be seen that The Seals Test produced a significant main effect for the cognitive training group (F (1,32) = 13.991). This result unequivocally asserted that the main treatment group displayed a significant difference on pre and

Table 13.1 Ratios of planned contrasts

Variable 1: F (1,32) ratios for planned contrasts					
Variable	A1	A2	B	A1B	A2B
Maze errors	0.440	0.127	0.099	0.019	0.766
Maze number	5.021	0.055	2.654	0.027	0.009
Maze time	0.107	0.028	12.583	0.370	0.010
NV memory	1.079	0.011	0.009	1.097	2.035
Verbal memory	0.070	1.271	1.813	0.498	1.241
Delayed memory	0.120	0.000	1.986	0.004	0.692
Metacognitive	1.231	0.910	2.206	0.513	0.366
Emotional	0.108	1.063	0.897	0.417	1.017
WIAT spelling	0.169	0.148	0.723	2.795	0.134
WIAT reading	0.443	0.153	0.544	2.680	1.104
WIAT mathematics	2.060	0.400	0.058	1.748	0.042
WCST correct	0.031	0.195	1.236	1.467	0.059
WCST persev	2.876	0.138	0.093	0.042	0.157
WCST time	0.169	0.148	0.723	2.795	0.134
Seals Test	0.181	1.269	12.727*	13.991*	1.495

*Significant at Bonferroni adjusted level

Table 13.2 Mean scores for the Seals Test

Group	Pre-test	Post-test
Cognitive training	60.5	78.786
Standard deviation	19.05	12.386
Placebo	68.182	73.727
Standard deviation	14.627	13.146
Control	65	63.9
Standard deviation	12.884	13.254

Table 13.3 Difference in raw scores for The Seals Test

Groups	Difference bet. pre and post-testing
Cognitive training	−18.286
Placebo	1.100
Control	−5.546

post-testing in comparison to the difference in pre and post-testing for either the placebo group or the control group.

An examination of mean scores and standard deviations on pre and post-testing on The Seals Test for the three groups is detailed in Table 13.2.

An examination of the difference in group raw scores on pre and post-testing on The Seals Test is contained in Table 13.3. The scores were based on pre-test minus post-test.

The size of the difference between pre and post-testing between the two control groups and the treatment group was 16.063, based on averaging the difference between the control groups and subtracting this from the treatment group difference. When this overall difference was converted to a standard score, the size of the treatment difference was 0.994, equivalent to 1 standard deviation. By conventional standards this difference was significant.

Austin Maze

The results of Table 13.1 also indicate that there was a significant difference between pre- and post-testing operating for the Austin Maze time taken. This difference was observable across the three subject groups.

Functional Executive Scale (FES)

It was hypothesised that there would be a significant improvement between pre- and post-testing on teacher observations on the functional executive scale. Table 13.4 details the mean pre- and post-test results for the three groups.

Table 13.4 Pre and post-test scores for functional executive scale

Group	Pre-test mean scores	Post-test mean scores	Improvement
Cognitive training	1.962	2.091	0.514
Standard deviation	0.251	0.237	
Placebo	1.923	2.018	0.475
Standard deviation	0.200	0.238	
Control	1.824	1.836	0.033
Standard deviation	0.356	0.466	

The results from Table 13.4 indicate that the size of the difference between pre- and post-testing for the three groups was in the expected direction but did not reach significance. The improvement in scores for the cognitive training group was more than 0.5 standard deviations, a result which was an acceptable outcome. The gain in standard deviations for the other groups was 0.48 for the placebo group and 0.03 for the control group.

Self-Monitoring Charts

All subjects in the CTG completed a self-monitoring chart indicating the percentage of time they believed they were applying the cognitive strategies to their school work and completing certain on-task behaviours. These charts recorded the information for 3 consecutive days on three separate working weeks during the intervention period. The first probe was taken at the beginning of the intervention period, the second probe after 5 weeks and the third probe after 10 weeks. The results are detailed in Table 13.5.

Significant improvement is evident in the substantial increase in percentage use of the strategies from a mean of 29% at the first probe, 42.75% at the second probe and 70.25% at the third probe.

Discussion

The results of this study indicated that there was a significant improvement on a measure of executive function for adolescents with moderate to severe traumatic brain injuries who were provided direct instruction on the use of a problem solving plan. The results of an ANOVA demonstrated that this improvement did not occur with a matched group of subjects who received non-executive function intervention or no intervention.

Given the stringent Bonferroni correction for significance of test results, the present finding was considered to be a valid outcome. The present finding was consistent with the hypothesis that neuropsychological measures assessing executive function were sensitive to improvements gained following intervention programs

Table 13.5 Data from 8 Cognitive Training subjects detailing % of time they were using the HBMPC plan in class

Beginning of intervention	After 5 weeks	After 10 weeks
0	0	25
50	67	60
75	83	90
7	50	100
35	37	36
42	60	88
0	0	75
23	45	88
Mean score = 29%	**Mean score = 42.75%**	**Mean score = 70.25%**

for adolescents with traumatic brain injuries. The present result was also consistent with previous studies involving problem-solving intervention programs with subjects with traumatic brain injuries.

In their study Von Cramon (1991) found a significant and positive pre- and post-test performance on the Tower of Hanoi. The current study was consistent with the Von Cramon result given that The Seals Test was an adaptation of the Tower of Hanoi.

The current results also revealed a strong trend in teacher-reported behaviours mediated by executive functions from the direct intervention group with an improvement on pre- and post-testing of more than 0.5 standard deviations. The results suggested that teachers were aware of a notable improvement in executive functioning only from the cognitive training group following the intervention. In particular, it was noted that the executive function behaviours that were rated as having significantly improved following the intervention were those that related to metacognitive functioning: attending, working independently, following through with instructions and using planning and organisational strategies.

The positive result on a functional measure was considered a critical outcome of this study. It demonstrated that not only would the CTG intervention produce significant improvement as measured by clinical tests but that the results would be observable by those working with the subjects on a day-to-day basis. It was considered that the results obtained by teacher ratings of metacognitive functions provided strong evidence that teachers had observed noticeable and positive changes in metacognitive functioning from the CTG subjects.

Another notable result was the significant improvement in time to complete the Austin Maze from the cognitive training group following the intervention. This result would suggest that, following the direct intervention, the CTG were significantly more efficient in completing the mazes possibly as a result of employing more efficient strategies.

The results of the self-monitoring probes by the CTG also indicated a perceived positive outcome in some school behaviours. The behaviour "I remembered what I had to do in class today" did display a positive improvement over the period of intervention. At the beginning of the intervention, the mean percentage of time engaged in this behaviour was 69% which increased to 85% after 5 weeks and then 88% at the end of 10 weeks. This behaviour was one that was not directly taught as part of the CTG intervention but was seen as a positive outcome of the process. Working memory was a by-product of the metacognitive strategy.

The CTG were taught to use a generic problem solving strategy that could be applied across curriculum content. In particular, CTG subjects were shown how the generic strategy could be applied to real-world problems that students faced every day in the classroom. It was argued that this approach obviated the need to teach specifically to generalisation, an issue in previous studies (Rabbit 1997). The CTG were provided opportunities in the intervention phase to practise the metacognitive strategy across the curriculum using their homework exercises and then to self-monitor their efforts in applying the strategy in the classroom.

Wood and Fussey (1994) observed that the need for rehabilitation subjects to apply, in real-life situations, the skills learned in therapy had been long recognised by the rehabilitation community.

A limitation of the study was the small numbers involved. In addition, a follow-up study could have been valuable in determining whether the cognitive training group continued to use the HBMPC problem solving plan following the intervention phase and that gains were maintained. In the real world, though, teachers would have been aware of the problem-solving strategy and encouraged their students to continue to employ HBMPC.

Nonetheless, the current study did provide some efficacy for the use of metacognitive strategies in general and the Hairy Bikie metacognitive strategy in particular.

References

Bird, K. (1998). *Psy 32 for windows*. University of NSW.

Bogan, J. (Baron Levi). (1994). *The assessment of executive function in children: A developmental perspective*. PhD thesis. University of New England.

Cicerone, J. D., & Wood, J. C. (1987). Planning disorder after closed head injury: A case study. *Archives of Physical and Medical Rehabilitation, 68*, 111–115.

Nelson, H. E. (1976). A modified card sorting test sensitive to frontal lobe deficits. *Cortex, 12*, 313–324.

Rabbit, P. (1997). Methodologies and models in the study of executive function. In P. Rabbit (Ed.), *Methodology of frontal and executive function*. East Sussex: Psychology Press Publishers.

Reynolds, C., & Bigler, E. D. (1994). *Test of memory and learning*. Austin, TX: Pro-ed.

Von Cramon, D. Y., et al. (1991). Problem solving deficits in brain injured patients: A therapeutic approach. *Neuropsychological Rehabilitation, 1*, 45–64.

Walsh, K. (1985). *Understanding brain damage: A primer of neuropsychological evaluation*. Edinburgh: Churchill Livingston.

Wechsler, D. (1992). *Wechsler individual achievement test*. Psychological Corporation.

Wood, R., & Fussey, I. (1994). *Cognitive rehabilitation in perspective*. Hove, UK: Lawrence Erlbaum Associates Publishers.

Glossary

Cogmed method Cogmed is a software-based intervention entailing different visuospatial and verbal tasks that systematically challenge the working memory capacity during a 5–10-week training period. The exercises are performed on a computer.

Cortical thickness Is a brain morphometric measure used to describe the combined thickness of the layers of the cerebral cortex in mammalian brains, either in local terms or as a global average for the entire brain.

Dendrite Short-branched extension of a nerve cell, along which impulses received from other cells at synapses are transmitted to the cell body.

Dorsolateral prefrontal cortex Is an area in the prefrontal cortex of the brain of humans and non-human primates. It is one of the most recently derived parts of the human brain. It undergoes a prolonged period of maturation which lasts until adulthood. The dorsolateral prefrontal cortex is not an anatomical structure, but rather a functional one. It lies in the middle frontal gyrus of humans.

Glasgow Coma Scale Is a neurological scale which aims to give a reliable and objective way of recording the state of a person's consciousness for initial as well as subsequent assessment. A person is assessed against the criteria of the scale, and the resulting points give a person's score between 3 (indicating deep unconsciousness) and 15 (more widely used, modified or revised scale).

Glial activity The four main functions of glial cells are to surround neurons and hold them in place, to supply nutrients and oxygen to neurons, to insulate one neuron from another and to destroy and remove the carcasses of dead neurons (clean up).

Gyrus A gyrus is a ridge on the cerebral cortex. It is generally surrounded by one or more sulci. Gyri and sulci create the folded appearance of the brain in humans and other mammals.

Korsakoff's syndrome Is an amnestic disorder caused by thiamine (vitamin B1) deficiency associated with prolonged ingestion of alcohol

Medial prefrontal cortex Is the large anterior or frontal lobes of the human brain and seems to be the centre of higher cognitive functions. Functional magnetic

J. Baron Levi, *The Hairy Bikie and Other Metacognitive Strategies*,
https://doi.org/10.1007/978-3-030-46618-3

resonance imaging examinations of activity in these parts of the brain suggest that they are the centre of processing of social information and memory functions related to the past and the making of long-term decisions for the future.

Orbito-frontal prefrontal cortex The orbitofrontal cortex refers to the smallest part of the frontal lobe in the brain. Functional MRIs allow doctors to track blood flow in the orbitofrontal cortex. Brain activity tests show that the orbito-frontal cortex is highly active during anything that involves learning new information.

Prefrontal cortex The prefrontal cortex is the cerebral cortex which is the grey matter that covers the front part of the frontal lobe.

Synapse A synapse is a structure that permits a neuron (or nerve cell) to pass an electrical or chemical signal to another neuron or to the target effector cell.

Ventral attention network Is one of two sensory orienting systems in the human brain, the other being the dorsal attention network (DAN). Its main function is to reorient attention towards salient stimuli.

Index

J. Baron Levi, *The Hairy Bikie and Other Metacognitive Strategies*,
https://doi.org/10.1007/978-3-030-46618-3

MIX
Papier aus verantwortungsvollen Quellen
Paper from responsible sources
FSC® C105338

If you have any concerns about our products, you can contact us on
ProductSafety@springernature.com

In case Publisher is established outside the EU, the EU authorized representative is:
Springer Nature Customer Service Center GmbH
Europaplatz 3, 69115 Heidelberg, Germany

Printed by Libri Plureos GmbH
in Hamburg, Germany